Medical Language
Instant
Translator

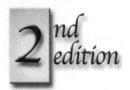

2 nd edition

Davi-Ellen Chabner, B.A., M.A.T.

Medical Language
Instant
Translator

2nd edition

SAUNDERS

An Imprint of Elsevier

610
Ch

SAUNDERS

An Imprint of Elsevier

11830 Westline Industrial Drive
St. Louis, Missouri 63146

MEDICAL LANGUAGE INSTANT TRANSLATOR   0-7216-0366-1

Copyright © 2004, Elsevier (USA). All rights reserved.

NOTICE

Medical terminology is an ever-changing field. Standard safety precautions must be followed, but as new research and clinical experience broaden our knowledge, changes in treatment and drug therapy may become necessary or appropriate. Readers are advised to check the most current product information provided by the manufacturer of each drug to be administered to verify the recommended dose, the method and duration of administration, and contraindications. It is the responsibility of the licensed prescriber, relying on experience and knowledge of the patient, to determine dosages and the best treatment for each individual patient. Neither the publisher nor the author assumes any liability for any injury and/or damage to persons or property arising form this publication.

Previous edition copyrighted 2001.

International Standard Book Number 0-7216-0366-1

Acquisitions Editor: Jeanne Wilke
Developmental Editor: Becky Swisher
Publishing Services Manager: Pat Joiner
Project Manager: Gena Magouirk
Designer: Ellen Zanolle

Printed in USA.

Last digit is the print number: 9 8 7 6 5 4 3 2

Welcome

This *Medical Language Instant Translator* will provide quick access to useful, medically related information for both laypersons and students entering the health-related professions. Today we are increasingly exposed to medical terminology, whether it be at the doctor's office, on the Internet, or in the media. Analyzing and understanding these terms allows us to participate in important issues affecting our society as well as to make better decisions about our own health.

Using this handy pocket-sized book, you will be able to:

- Decipher complicated medical terms by recognizing and finding the meanings of individual word parts;
- Distinguish between commonly misunderstood medical terms;
- Access information on medical abbreviations, symbols, acronyms, and professional designations;
- Easily access surgical terminology;
- Understand the definitions of commonly used diagnostic tests and procedures;
- Identify the top 100 prescription drugs and their uses;
- Interpret the significance of common blood tests;
- Visualize the location of many organs and body structures with full-color illustrations.

Although this *Instant Translator* dovetails with information in both my books, *The Language of Medicine* and *Medical Terminology: A Short Course*, all students of the medical language can benefit from it. Please let me know how the *Instant Translator* works for you, and have fun using it!

Davi-Ellen Chabner
MedDavi@aol.com

Contents

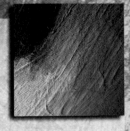

Part 3
BODY SYSTEMS ILLUSTRATIONS

Medical Language Instant Translator

2nd edition

part

THE LANGUAGE
OF MEDICINE

How to Analyze Medical Terms*

Studying medical terminology is very similar to learning a new language. At first the words sound strange and complicated, although they may stand for commonly known English terms. For example, the term **otalgia** means "ear ache," and an **ophthalmologist** is an "eye doctor."

Your first job in learning the language is to understand how to divide words into their component parts. Logically most terms, whether complex or simple, can be broken down into basic parts and then understood. For example, consider the following term:

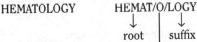

HEMATOLOGY   HEMAT/O/LOGY

root   suffix

combining vowel

The **root** is the *foundation of the word.* All medical terms have one or more roots. The root **hemat** means **blood.**

The **suffix** is the *word ending.* All medical terms have a suffix. The suffix **-logy** means **study of.**

The **combining vowel** (usually o) *links the root to the suffix or the root to another root.* A combining vowel has no meaning of its own; it only joins one word part to another.

It is useful to read the meaning of medical terms starting from the suffix and moving back to the beginning of the term. Thus, the term **hematology** means **study of blood.**

---

*From Chabner D-E: The Language of Medicine, 7th ed. Philadelphia, WB Saunders, 2004.

Here is another familiar medical term:

ELECTROCARDIOGRAM   ELECTR/O/CARDI/O/GRAM

↓   ↓   ↓
root   root   suffix

combining vowel

The root **electr** means **electricity.**
The root **cardi** means **heart.**
The suffix **-gram** means **record.**
The entire word means **record of the electricity in the heart.**

Notice that there are two combining vowels in this term. They link the two roots **(electr and cardi)** as well as the root **(cardi)** and suffix **(-gram).**

Try another term:

GASTRITIS   GASTR/ITIS

↓   ↓
root   suffix

The root **gastr** means **stomach.**
The suffix **-itis** means **inflammation.**

The entire word, reading from the end of the term (suffix) to the beginning, means **inflammation of the stomach.**

Note that the combining vowel, o, is missing in this term. This is because the suffix, **-itis,** begins with a vowel. The combining vowel is dropped before a suffix that begins with a vowel. It is retained, however, between two roots, even if the second root begins with a vowel. Consider the following term:

GASTROENTEROLOGY   GASTR/O/ENTER/O/LOGY

↓   ↓   ↓
root   root   suffix

combining vowel

The root **gastr** means **stomach.**
The root **enter** means **intestines.**
The suffix **-logy** means **study of.**
The entire term means **study of the stomach and intestines.**

Notice that the combining vowel is used between **gastr** and **enter,** even though the second root, **enter,** begins with a vowel. When a term contains two or more roots related to parts of the body, anatomical position often determines which root goes before the other. For example, the stomach receives food first, before the small intestine, thus, **gastroenteritis,** not enterogastritis.

In summary, remember three general rules:

1. Read the meaning of medical terms from the suffix back to the beginning of the term and across.
2. Drop the combining vowel (usually o) before a suffix beginning with a vowel: **gastritis,** *not* **gastroitis.**
3. Keep the combining vowel between two roots: **gastroenterology,** *not* **gastrenterology.**

In addition to the root, suffix, and combining vowel, two other word parts are commonly found in medical terms. These are the **combining form** and **prefix.** The combining form is simply the root plus the combining vowel. For example, you are already familiar with the following combining forms and their meanings:

HEMAT/O   means   **blood**

↗   ↗

root + combining vowel = COMBINING FORM

GASTR/O   means   **stomach**

↗   ↗

root + combining vowel = COMBINING FORM

Combining forms are used with many different suffixes. Remembering the exact meaning of a combining form will help you understand different medical terms.

The **prefix** is a small part that is attached to the *beginning of a term.* Not all medical terms contain prefixes, but the prefix can have an important influence on meaning. Consider the following examples:

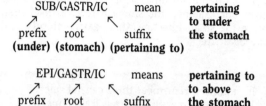

In summary, the important elements of medical terms are:
1. **Root:** foundation of the term
2. **Suffix:** word ending
3. **Prefix:** word beginning
4. **Combining vowel:** vowel (usually o) that links the root to the suffix or the root to another root
5. **Combining form:** combination of the root and the combining vowel

Glossary of Word Parts Used in Medical Terminology*

Medical Word Parts—English

Combining Form, Prefix, or Suffix	Meaning
a-, an-	no; not; without
ab-	away from
abdomin/o	abdomen
-ac	pertaining to
acanth/o	spiny; thorny
acetabul/o	acetabulum (hip socket)
acous/o	hearing
acr/o	extremities; top; extreme point
acromi/o	acromion (extension of shoulder bone)
actin/o	light
acu/o	sharp; severe; sudden
-acusis	hearing
ad-	toward
aden/o	gland
adenoid/o	adenoids
adip/o	fat
adren/o	adrenal gland
adrenal/o	adrenal gland
aer/o	air
af-	toward
agglutin/o	clumping; sticking together

Chart continued on following page

*From Chabner D-E: The Language of Medicine, 7th ed. Philadelphia, WB Saunders, 2004.

Medical Word Parts—English *Continued*

Combining Form, Prefix, or Suffix	Meaning
-agon	to assemble, gather
agora-	marketplace
-agra	excessive pain
-al	pertaining to
alb/o	white
albin/o	white
albumin/o	albumin (protein)
alges/o	sensitivity to pain
-algesia	sensitivity to pain
-algia	pain
all/o	other
alveol/o	alveolus; air sac; small sac
ambly/o	dim; dull
-amine	nitrogen compound
amni/o	amnion (sac surrounding the embryo)
amyl/o	starch
an/o	anus
-an	pertaining to
ana-	up; apart; backward; again, anew
andr/o	male
aneurysm/o	aneurysm (widened blood vessel)
angi/o	vessel (blood)
anis/o	unequal
ankyl/o	stiff
ante-	before; forward
anter/o	front
anthrac/o	coal
anthr/o	antrum of the stomach
anti-	against
anxi/o	uneasy; anxious
aort/o	aorta (largest artery)
-apheresis	removal
aphth/o	ulcer
apo-	off, away
aponeur/o	aponeurosis (type of tendon)

Medical Word Parts—English *Continued*

Combining Form, Prefix, or Suffix	Meaning
append/o	appendix
appendic/o	appendix
aque/o	water
-ar	pertaining to
-arche	beginning
arter/o	artery
arteri/o	artery
arteriol/o	arteriole (small artery)
arthr/o	joint
-arthria	articulate (speak distinctly)
articul/o	joint
-ary	pertaining to
asbest/o	asbestos
-ase	enzyme
-asthenia	lack of strength
atel/o	incomplete
ather/o	plaque (fatty substance)
-ation	process; condition
atri/o	atrium (upper heart chamber)
audi/o	hearing
audit/o	hearing
aur/o	ear
auricul/o	ear
auto-	self, own
axill/o	armpit
azot/o	urea; nitrogen
bacill/o	bacilli (bacteria)
bacteri/o	bacteria
balan/o	glans penis
bar/o	pressure; weight
bartholin/o	Bartholin glands
bas/o	base; opposite of acid
bi-	two

Chart continued on following page

Medical Word Parts—English *Continued*

Combining Form, Prefix, or Suffix	Meaning
bi/o	life
bil/i	bile; gall
bilirubin/o	bilirubin
-blast	embryonic; immature
-blastoma	immature tumor (cells)
blephar/o	eyelid
bol/o	cast; throw
brachi/o	arm
brachy-	short
brady-	slow
bronch/o	bronchial tube
bronchi/o	bronchial tube
bronchiol/o	bronchiole
bucc/o	cheek
bunion/o	bunion
burs/o	bursa (sac of fluid near joints)
byssin/o	cotton dust
cac/o	bad
calc/o	calcium
calcane/o	calcaneus (heel bone)
calci/o	calcium
cali/o	calyx
calic/o	calyx
capillar/o	capillary (tiniest blood vessel)
capn/o	carbon dioxide
-capnia	carbon dioxide
carcin/o	cancerous; cancer
cardi/o	heart
carp/o	wrist bones (carpals)
cata-	down
caud/o	tail; lower part of body
caus/o	burn; burning
cauter/o	heat; burn

Medical Word Parts—English *Continued*

Combining Form, Prefix, or Suffix	Meaning
cec/o	cecum (first part of the colon)
-cele	hernia
celi/o	belly; abdomen
-centesis	surgical puncture to remove fluid
cephal/o	head
cerebell/o	cerebellum (posterior part of the brain)
cerebr/o	cerebrum (largest part of the brain)
cerumin/o	cerumen
cervic/o	neck; cervix (neck of uterus)
-chalasia	relaxation
-chalasis	relaxation
cheil/o	lip
chem/o	drug; chemical
-chezia	defecation; elimination of wastes
chir/o	hand
chlor/o	green
chlorhydr/o	hydrochloric acid
chol/e	bile; gall
cholangi/o	bile vessel
cholecyst/o	gallbladder
choledoch/o	common bile duct
cholesterol/o	cholesterol
chondr/o	cartilage
chore/o	dance
chori/o	chorion (outermost membrane of the fetus)
chorion/o	chorion
choroid/o	choroid layer of eye
chrom/o	color
chron/o	time
chym/o	to pour
cib/o	meal
-cidal	pertaining to killing

Chart continued on following page

Medical Word Parts—English *Continued*

Combining Form, Prefix, or Suffix	Meaning
-cide	killing
cine/o	movement
cirrh/o	orange-yellow
cis/o	to cut
-clasis	to break
-clast	to break
claustr/o	enclosed space
clavicul/o	clavicle (collar bone)
-clysis	irrigation; washing
coagul/o	coagulation (clotting)
-coccus (-cocci, pl.)	berry-shaped bacterium
coccyg/o	coccyx (tailbone)
cochle/o	cochlea (inner part of ear)
col/o	colon (large intestine)
coll/a	glue
colon/o	colon (large intestine)
colp/o	vagina
comat/o	deep sleep
comi/o	to care for
con-	together, with
coni/o	dust
conjunctiv/o	conjunctiva (lines the eyelids)
-constriction	narrowing
contra-	against; opposite
cor/o	pupil
core/o	pupil
corne/o	cornea
coron/o	heart
corpor/o	body
cortic/o	cortex; outer region
cost/o	rib
crani/o	skull
cras/o	mixture; temperament
crin/o	secrete

Medical Word Parts—English *Continued*

Combining Form, Prefix, or Suffix	Meaning
-crine	secrete; separate
-crit	to separate
cry/o	cold
crypt/o	hidden
culd/o	cul-de-sac
-cusis	hearing
cutane/o	skin
cyan/o	blue
cycl/o	ciliary body of eye; cycle; circle
-cyesis	pregnancy
cyst/o	urinary bladder; cyst; sac of fluid
cyt/o	cell
-cyte	cell
-cytosis	condition of cells; slight increase in numbers
dacry/o	tear
dacryoaden/o	tear gland
dacryocyst/o	tear sac; lacrimal sac
dactyl/o	fingers; toes
de-	lack of; down; less; removal of
dem/o	people
dent/i	tooth
derm/o	skin
-derma	skin
dermat/o	skin
desicc/o	drying
-desis	to bind, tie together
dia-	complete; through
diaphor/o	sweat
-dilation	widening; stretching; expanding
dipl/o	double
dips/o	thirst

Chart continued on following page

Medical Word Parts—English *Continued*

Combining Form, Prefix, or Suffix	Meaning
dist/o	far; distant
dors/o	back (of body)
dorsi-	back
-dote	to give
-drome	to run
duct/o	to lead, carry
duoden/o	duodenum
dur/o	dura mater
-dynia	pain
dys-	bad; painful; difficult; abnormal
-eal	pertaining to
ec-	out; outside
echo-	reflected sound
-ectasia	stretching; dilation; expansion
-ectasis	stretching; dilation; expansion
ecto-	out; outside
-ectomy	removal; excision; resection
-edema	swelling
-elasma	flat plate
electr/o	electricity
em-	in
-ema	condition
-emesis	vomiting
-emia	blood condition
-emic	pertaining to blood condition
emmetr/o	in due measure
en-	in; within
encephal/o	brain
endo-	in; within
enter/o	intestines (usually small intestine)
eosin/o	red; rosy; dawn-colored
epi-	above; upon; on
epididym/o	epididymis
epiglott/o	epiglottis

Medical Word Parts—English *Continued*

Combining Form, Prefix, or Suffix	Meaning
episi/o	vulva (external female genitalia)
epitheli/o	skin; epithelium
equin/o	horse
-er	one who
erg/o	work
erythem/o	flushed; redness
erythr/o	red
-esis	condition
eso-	inward
esophag/o	esophagus
esthes/o	nervous sensation (feeling)
esthesi/o	nervous sensation
-esthesia	nervous sensation
estr/o	female
ethm/o	sieve
eti/o	cause
eu-	good; normal
-eurysm	widening
ex-	out; away from
exanthemat/o	rash
exo-	out; away from
extra-	outside
faci/o	face
fasci/o	fascia (membrane supporting muscles)
femor/o	femur (thigh bone)
-ferent	to carry
fibr/o	fiber
fibros/o	fibrous connective tissue
fibul/o	fibula
-fication	process of making
-fida	split
flex/o	to bend

Chart continued on following page

Medical Word Parts—English *Continued*

Combining Form, Prefix, or Suffix	Meaning
fluor/o	luminous
follicul/o	follicle; small sac
-form	resembling; in the shape of
fung/i	fungus; mushroom
furc/o	forking; branching
-fusion	to pour; to come together
galact/o	milk
ganglion/o	ganglion; collection of nerve cell bodies
gastr/o	stomach
-gen	producing; forming
-genesis	producing; forming
-genic	produced by or in
ger/o	old age
gest/o	pregnancy
gester/o	pregnancy
gingiv/o	gum
glauc/o	gray
gli/o	glue; neuroglial tissue (supportive tissue of nervous system)
-globin	protein
-globulin	protein
glomerul/o	glomerulus
gloss/o	tongue
gluc/o	glucose; sugar
glyc/o	glucose; sugar
glycogen/o	glycogen; animal starch
glycos/o	glucose; sugar
gnos/o	knowledge
gon/o	seed
gonad/o	sex glands
goni/o	angle
-grade	to go
-gram	record

Medical Word Parts—English *Continued*

Combining Form, Prefix, or Suffix	Meaning
granul/o	granule(s)
-graph	instrument for recording
-graphy	process of recording
gravid/o	pregnancy
-gravida	pregnant woman
gynec/o	woman; female
hallucin/o	hallucination
hem/o	blood
hemat/o	blood
hemi-	half
hemoglobin/o	hemoglobin
hepat/o	liver
herni/o	hernia
-hexia	habit
hidr/o	sweat
hist/o	tissue
histi/o	tissue
home/o	sameness; unchanging; constant
hormon/o	hormone
humer/o	humerus (upper arm bone)
hydr/o	water
hyper-	above; excessive
hypn/o	sleep
hypo-	deficient; below; under; less than normal
hypophys/o	pituitary gland
hyster/o	uterus; womb
-ia	condition
-iac	pertaining to
-iasis	abnormal condition

Chart continued on following page

Medical Word Parts—English *Continued*

Combining Form, Prefix, or Suffix	Meaning
iatr/o	physician; treatment
-ic	pertaining to
-ical	pertaining to
ichthy/o	dry; scaly
-icle	small
idi/o	unknown; individual; distinct
ile/o	ileum (part of small intestine)
ili/o	ilium (part of hip bone)
immun/o	immune; protection; safe
in-	in; into; not
-in, -ine	a substance
-ine	pertaining to
infra-	below; inferior to; beneath
inguin/o	groin
insulin/o	insulin (pancreatic hormone)
inter-	between
intra-	within; into
iod/o	iodine
ion/o	ion; to wander
-ion	process
-ior	pertaining to
ipsi-	same
ir-	in
ir/o	iris (colored portion of eye)
irid/o	iris (colored portion of eye)
is/o	same; equal
isch/o	to hold back; back
ischi/o	ischium (part of hip bone)
-ism	process; condition
-ist	specialist
-itis	inflammation
-ium	structure; tissue
jaund/o	yellow
jejun/o	jejunum

Medical Word Parts—English *Continued*

Combining Form, Prefix, or Suffix	Meaning
kal/i	potassium
kary/o	nucleus
kerat/o	horny, hard; cornea
kern-	nucleus (collection of nerve cells in the brain)
ket/o	ketones; acetones
keton/o	ketones; acetones
kines/o	movement
kinesi/o	movement
-kinesia	movement
-kinesis	movement
klept/o	to steal
kyph/o	humpback
labi/o	lip
lacrim/o	tear; tear duct; lacrimal duct
lact/o	milk
lamin/o	lamina (part of vertebral arch)
lapar/o	abdominal wall; abdomen
-lapse	to slide, fall, sag
laryng/o	larynx (voice box)
later/o	side
leiomy/o	smooth (visceral) muscle
-lemma	sheath, covering
-lepsy	seizure
lept/o	thin, slender
-leptic	to seize, take hold of
leth/o	death
leuk/o	white
lute/o	yellow
lex/o	word; phrase
-lexia	word; phrase
ligament/o	ligament
lingu/o	tongue

Chart continued on following page

Medical Word Parts—English *Continued*

Combining Form, Prefix, or Suffix	Meaning
lip/o	fat; lipid
-listhesis	slipping
lith/o	stone; calculus
-lithiasis	condition of stones
-lithotomy	incision (for removal) of a stone
lob/o	lobe
log/o	study of
-logy	study of
lord/o	curve; swayback
-lucent	to shine
lumb/o	lower back; loin
lute/o	yellow
lux/o	to slide
lymph/o	lymph
lymphaden/o	lymph gland (node)
lymphangi/o	lymph vessel
-lysis	breakdown; separation; destruction; loosening
-lytic	to reduce, destroy; separate; break down
macro-	large
mal-	bad
-malacia	softening
malleol/o	malleolus
mamm/o	breast
mandibul/o	mandible (lower jaw bone)
-mania	obsessive preoccupation
mast/o	breast
mastoid/o	mastoid process (behind the ear)
maxill/o	maxilla (upper jaw bone)
meat/o	meatus (opening)
medi/o	middle
mediastin/o	mediastinum

Medical Word Parts—English *Continued*

Combining Form, Prefix, or Suffix	Meaning
medull/o	medulla (inner section); middle; soft, marrow
mega-	large
-megaly	enlargement
melan/o	black
men/o	menses; menstruation
mening/o	meninges (membranes covering the spinal cord and brain)
meningi/o	meninges
ment/o	mind; chin
meso-	middle
meta-	change; beyond
metacarp/o	metacarpals (hand bones)
metatars/o	metatarsals (foot bones)
-meter	measure
metr/o	uterus (womb); measure
metri/o	uterus (womb)
mi/o	smaller; less
micro-	small
-mimetic	mimic; copy
-mission	to send
mon/o	one; single
morph/o	shape; form
mort/o	death
-mortem	death
-motor	movement
muc/o	mucus
mucos/o	mucous membrane (mucosa)
multi-	many
mut/a	genetic change
mutagen/o	causing genetic change
my/o	muscle
myc/o	fungus
mydr/o	wide

Chart continued on following page

Medical Word Parts—English *Continued*

Combining Form, Prefix, or Suffix	Meaning
myel/o	spinal cord; bone marrow
myocardi/o	myocardium (heart muscle)
myom/o	muscle tumor
myos/o	muscle
myring/o	tympanic membrane (eardrum)
myx/o	mucus
narc/o	numbness; stupor; sleep
nas/o	nose
nat/i	birth
natr/o	sodium
necr/o	death
nect/o	to bind, tie, connect
neo-	new
nephr/o	kidney
neur/o	nerve
neutr/o	neither; neutral
nid/o	nest
noct/i	night
norm/o	rule; order
nos/o	disease
nucle/o	nucleus
nulli-	none
nyct/o	night
obstetr/o	midwife
ocul/o	eye
odont/o	tooth
odyn/o	pain
-oid	resembling
-ole	little; small
olecran/o	olecranon (elbow)
olig/o	scanty

Medical Word Parts—English *Continued*

Combining Form, Prefix, or Suffix	Meaning
om/o	shoulder
-oma	tumor; mass; fluid collection
omphal/o	umbilicus (navel)
onc/o	tumor
-one	hormone
onych/o	nail (of fingers or toes)
o/o	egg
oophor/o	ovary
-opaque	obscure
ophthalm/o	eye
-opia	vision
-opsia	vision
-opsy	view of
opt/o	eye; vision
optic/o	eye; vision
-or	one who
or/o	mouth
orch/o	testis
orchi/o	testis
orchid/o	testis
-orexia	appetite
orth/o	straight
-ose	full of; pertaining to; sugar
-osis	condition, usually abnormal
-osmia	smell
ossicul/o	ossicle (small bone)
oste/o	bone
-ostosis	condition of bone
ot/o	ear
-otia	ear condition
-ous	pertaining to
ov/o	egg
ovari/o	ovary
ovul/o	egg

Chart continued on following page

Medical Word Parts—English *Continued*

Combining Form, Prefix, or Suffix	Meaning
ox/o	oxygen
-oxia	oxygen
oxy-	swift; sharp; acid
oxysm/o	sudden
pachy-	heavy; thick
palat/o	palate (roof of the mouth)
palpebr/o	eyelid
pan-	all
pancreat/o	pancreas
papill/o	nipple-like; optic disc (disk)
par-	other than; abnormal
para-	near; beside; abnormal; apart from; along the side of
-para	to bear, bring forth (live births)
-parous	to bear, bring forth
parathyroid/o	parathyroid glands
-paresis	slight paralysis
-pareunia	sexual intercourse
-partum	birth; labor
patell/a	patella (kneecap)
patell/o	patella
path/o	disease
-pathy	disease; emotion
pector/o	chest
ped/o	child; foot
pelv/i	pelvic bone; hip
pend/o	to hang
-penia	deficiency
-pepsia	digestion
per-	through
peri-	surrounding
perine/o	perineum
peritone/o	peritoneum

Medical Word Parts—English *Continued*

Combining Form, Prefix, or Suffix	Meaning
perone/o	fibula
-pexy	fixation; to put in place
phac/o	lens of eye
phag/o	eat; swallow
-phage	eat; swallow
-phagia	eating; swallowing
phak/o	lens of eye
phalang/o	phalanges (fingers and toes)
phall/o	penis
pharmac/o	drug
pharmaceut/o	drug
pharyng/o	throat (pharynx)
phas/o	speech
-phasia	speech
phe/o	dusky; dark
-pheresis	removal
phil/o	like; love; attraction to
-phil	attraction for
-philia	attraction for
phim/o	muzzle
phleb/o	vein
phob/o	fear
-phobia	fear
phon/o	voice; sound
-phonia	voice; sound
-phor/o	to bear
-phoresis	carrying; transmission
-phoria	to bear, carry; feeling (mental state)
phot/o	light
phren/o	diaphragm; mind
-phthisis	wasting away
-phylaxis	protection
physi/o	nature; function
-physis	to grow

Chart continued on following page

Medical Word Parts—English *Continued*

Combining Form, Prefix, or Suffix	Meaning
phyt/o	plant
-phyte	plant
pil/o	hair
pineal/o	pineal gland
pituitar/o	pituitary gland
-plakia	plaque
plant/o	sole of the foot
plas/o	development; formation
-plasia	development; formation; growth
-plasm	formation
-plastic	pertaining to formation
-plasty	surgical repair
ple/o	more; many
-plegia	paralysis; palsy
-plegic	paralysis; palsy
pleur/o	pleura
plex/o	plexus; network (of nerves)
-pnea	breathing
pneum/o	lung; air; gas
pneumon/o	lung; air; gas
pod/o	foot
-poiesis	formation
-poietin	substance that forms
poikil/o	varied; irregular
pol/o	extreme
polio-	gray matter (of brain or spinal cord)
poly-	many; much
polyp/o	polyp; small growth
pont/o	pons (a part of the brain)
-porosis	condition of pores (spaces)
post-	after; behind
poster/o	back (of body); behind
-prandial	meal
-praxia	action
pre-	before; in front of
presby/o	old age

Medical Word Parts—English *Continued*

Combining Form, Prefix, or Suffix	Meaning
primi-	first
pro-	before; forward
proct/o	anus and rectum
pros-	before; forward
prostat/o	prostate gland
prot/o	first
prote/o	protein
proxim/o	near
prurit/o	itching
pseudo-	false
psych/o	mind
-ptosis	droop; sag; prolapse; fall
-ptysis	spitting
pub/o	pubis (anterior part of hip bone)
pulmon/o	lung
pupill/o	pupil (dark center of the eye)
purul/o	pus
py/o	pus
pyel/o	renal pelvis
pylor/o	pylorus; pyloric sphincter
pyr/o	fever; fire
pyret/o	fever
pyrex/o	fever
quadri-	four
rachi/o	spinal column; vertebrae
radi/o	x-rays; radioactivity; radius (lateral lower arm bone)
radicul/o	nerve root
re-	back; again; backward
rect/o	rectum
ren/o	kidney

Chart continued on following page

Medical Word Parts—English *Continued*

Combining Form, Prefix, or Suffix	Meaning
reticul/o	network
retin/o	retina
retro-	behind; back; backward
rhabdomy/o	striated (skeletal) muscle
rheumat/o	watery flow (in joints)
rhin/o	nose
rhytid/o	wrinkle
roentgen/o	x-rays
-rrhage	bursting forth (of blood)
-rrhagia	bursting forth (of blood)
-rrhaphy	suture
-rrhea	flow; discharge
- rrhexis	rupture
rrhythm/o	rhythm
sacr/o	sacrum
salping/o	fallopian tube; auditory (eustachian) tube
-salpinx	fallopian tube; oviduct
sarc/o	flesh (connective tissue)
scapul/o	scapula; shoulder blade
-schisis	to split
schiz/o	split
scint/i	spark
scirrh/o	hard
scler/o	sclera (white of the eye)
-sclerosis	hardening
scoli/o	crooked; bent
-scope	instrument for visual examination
-scopy	visual examination
scot/o	darkness
seb/o	sebum
sebace/o	sebum
sect/o	to cut
semi-	half

Medical Word Parts—English *Continued*

Combining Form, Prefix, or Suffix	Meaning
semin/i	semen; seed
seps/o	infection
sial/o	saliva
sialaden/o	salivary gland
sider/o	iron
sigmoid/o	sigmoid colon
silic/o	glass
sinus/o	sinus
-sis	state of; condition
-sol	solution
somat/o	body
-some	body
somn/o	sleep
-somnia	sleep
son/o	sound
-spadia	to tear, cut
-spasm	sudden contraction of muscles
sperm/o	spermatozoa; sperm cells
spermat/o	spermatozoa; sperm cells
sphen/o	wedge; sphenoid bone
spher/o	globe-shaped; round
sphygm/o	pulse
-sphyxia	pulse
spin/o	spine (backbone)
spir/o	to breathe
splanchn/o	viscera (internal organs)
splen/o	spleen
spondyl/o	vertebra (backbone)
squam/o	scale
-stalsis	contraction
staped/o	stapes (middle ear bone)
staphyl/o	clusters; uvula
-stasis	stop; control; place
-static	pertaining to stopping; controlling

Chart continued on following page

Medical Word Parts—English *Continued*

Combining Form, Prefix, or Suffix	Meaning
steat/o	fat, sebum
-stenosis	tightening; stricture
ster/o	solid structure; steroid
stere/o	solid; three-dimensional
stern/o	sternum (breastbone)
steth/o	chest
-sthenia	strength
-stitial	to set; pertaining to standing or positioned
stomat/o	mouth
-stomia	condition of the mouth
-stomy	new opening (to form a mouth)
strept/o	twisted chains
styl/o	pole or stake
sub-	under; below
submaxill/o	mandible (lower jaw bone)
-suppression	to stop
supra-	above, upper
sym-	together; with
syn-	together; with
syncop/o	to cut off, cut short; faint
syndesm/o	ligament
synov/o	synovia; synovial membrane; sheath around a tendon
syring/o	tube
tachy-	fast
tars/o	tarsus; hindfoot or ankle (7 bones between the foot and the leg)
tax/o	order; coordination
tel/o	complete
tele/o	distant
ten/o	tendon
tendin/o	tendon
-tension	pressure

Medical Word Parts—English *Continued*

Combining Form, Prefix, or Suffix	Meaning
terat/o	monster; malformed fetus
test/o	testis (testicle)
tetra-	four
thalam/o	thalamus
thalass/o	sea
the/o	put; place
thec/o	sheath
thel/o	nipple
therapeut/o	treatment
-therapy	treatment
therm/o	heat
thorac/o	chest
-thorax	chest; pleural cavity
thromb/o	clot
thym/o	thymus gland
-thymia	mind (condition of)
-thymic	pertaining to mind
thyr/o	thyroid gland; shield
thyroid/o	thyroid gland
tibi/o	tibia (shin bone)
-tic	pertaining to
toc/o	labor; birth
-tocia	labor; birth (condition of)
-tocin	labor; birth (a substance for)
tom/o	to cut
-tome	instrument to cut
-tomy	process of cutting
ton/o	tension
tone/o	to stretch
tonsill/o	tonsil
top/o	place; position; location
tox/o	poison
toxic/o	poison
trache/o	trachea (windpipe)
trans-	across; through

Chart continued on following page

Medical Word Parts—English *Continued*

Combining Form, Prefix, or Suffix	Meaning
-tresia	opening
tri-	three
trich/o	hair
trigon/o	trigone (area within the bladder)
-tripsy	to crush
troph/o	nourishment; development
-trophy	nourishment; development
-tropia	to turn
-tropic	turning
-tropin	stimulate; act on
tympan/o	tympanic membrane (eardrum); middle ear
-type	classification; picture
-ule	little; small
uln/o	ulna (medial lower arm bone)
ultra-	beyond; excess
-um	structure; tissue; thing
umbilic/o	umbilicus (navel)
ungu/o	nail
uni-	one
ur/o	urine; urinary tract
ureter/o	ureter
urethr/o	urethra
-uria	urination; condition of urine
urin/o	urine
-us	structure; thing
uter/o	uterus (womb)
uve/o	uvea, vascular layer of eye (iris, choroid, ciliary body)
uvul/o	uvula
vag/o	vagus nerve
vagin/o	vagina

Medical Word Parts—English *Continued*

Combining Form, Prefix, or Suffix	Meaning
valv/o	valve
valvul/o	valve
varic/o	varicose veins
vas/o	vessel; duct; vas deferens
vascul/o	vessel (blood)
ven/o	vein
vener/o	venereal (sexual contact)
ventr/o	belly side of body
ventricul/o	ventricle (of heart or brain)
venul/o	venule (small vein)
-verse	to turn
-version	to turn
vertebr/o	vertebra (backbone)
vesic/o	urinary bladder
vesicul/o	seminal vesicle
vestibul/o	vestibule of the inner ear
viscer/o	internal organs
vit/o	life
vitr/o	vitreous body (of the eye)
vitre/o	glass
viv/o	life
vol/o	to roll
vulv/o	vulva (female external genitalia)
xanth/o	yellow
xen/o	stranger
xer/o	dry
xiph/o	sword
-y	condition; process
zo/o	animal life

English—Medical Word Parts

Meaning	Combining Form, Prefix, or Suffix
abdomen	abdomin/o (use with -al, -centesis)
	celi/o (use with -ac)
	lapar/o (use with -scope, -scopy, -tomy)
abdominal wall	lapar/o
abnormal	dys-
	par-
	para-
abnormal condition	-iasis
	-osis
above	epi-
	hyper-
	supra-
acetabulum	acetabul/o
acetones	ket/o
	keton/o
acid	oxy-
acromion	acromi/o
across	trans-
action	-praxia
act on	-tropin
adrenal glands	adren/o
	adrenal/o
after	post-
again	ana-
	re-
against	anti-
	contra-
air	aer/o
	pneum/o
	pneumon/o
air sac	alveol/o
albumin	albumin/o
all	pan-
along the side of	para-

English—Medical Word Parts *Continued*

Meaning	Combining Form, Prefix, or Suffix
alveolus	alveol/o
amnion	amni/o
aneurysm	aneurysm/o
anew	ana-
angle	goni/o
animal life	zo/o
animal starch	glycogen/o
ankle	tars/o
anus	an/o
anus and rectum	proct/o
anxiety	anxi/o
apart	ana-
apart from	para-
appendix	append/o (use with -ectomy)
	appendic/o (use with -itis)
appetite	-orexia
arm	brachi/o
arm bone, lower, lateral	radi/o
arm bone, lower, medial	uln/o
arm bone, upper	humer/o
armpit	axill/o
arteriole	arteriol/o
artery	arter/o
	arteri/o
articulate (speak distinctly)	-arthria
asbestos	asbest/o
assemble	-agon
atrium	atri/o
attraction for	-phil
	-philia
attraction to	phil/o
auditory tube	salping/o

Chart continued on following page

English—Medical Word Parts *Continued*

Meaning	Combining Form, Prefix, or Suffix
away from	ab-
	apo-
	ex-
	exo-
back	re-
	retro-
back, lower	lumb/o
back portion of body	dorsi-
	dors/o
	poster/o
backbone	spin/o (use with -al)
	spondyl/o (use with -itis, -listhesis, -osis, -pathy)
	vertebr/o (use with -al)
backward	ana-
	retro-
bacteria	bacteri/o
bacterium (berry-shaped)	-coccus (-cocci, pl.)
bacilli (rod-shaped bacteria)	bacill/o
bad	cac/o
	dys-
	mal-
barrier	claustr/o
base (not acidic)	bas/o
bear (to)	-para
	-parous
	-phoria
	phor/o
before	ante-
	pre-
	pro-
	pros-

English—Medical Word Parts *Continued*

Meaning	Combining Form, Prefix, or Suffix
blood	hem/o (use with -dialysis, -globin, -lysis, -philia, -ptysis, -rrhage, -stasis, -stat)
	hemat/o (use with -crit, -emesis, -logist, -logy, -oma, -poiesis, -uria)
blood condition	-emia
	-emic
blood vessel	angi/o (use with -ectomy, -genesis, -gram, -graphy, -oma, -plasty, -spasm)
	vas/o (use with -constriction, -dilation, -motor)
	vascul/o (use with -ar, -itis)
blue	cyan/o
body	corpor/o
	somat/o
	-some
bone	oste/o
bone condition	-ostosis
bone marrow	myel/o
brain	encephal/o
	cerebr/o
branching	furc/o
break	-clasis
	-clast
breakdown	-lysis
breast	mamm/o (use with -ary, -gram, -graphy, -plasty)
	mast/o (use with -algia, -dynia, -ectomy, -itis)

English—Medical Word Parts *Continued*

Meaning	Combining Form, Prefix, or Suffix
beginning	-arche
behind	post-
	poster/o
	retro-
belly	celi/o
belly side of body	ventr/o
below, beneath	hypo-
	infra-
	sub-
bend (to)	flex/o
bent	ankyl/o
	scoli/o
beside	para-
between	inter-
beyond	hyper-
	meta-
	ultra-
bile	bil/i
	chol/e
bile vessel	cholangi/o
bilirubin	bilirubin/o
bind	-desis
	nect/o
birth	nat/i
	-partum
	toc/o
	-tocia
birth (substance for)	-tocin
births (live)	-para
black	anthrac/o, melan/o
bladder (urinary)	cyst/o (use with -ic, -itis, -cele, -gram, -scopy, -stomy, -tomy)
	vesic/o (use with -al)

Chart continued on following page

English—Medical Word Parts *Continued*

Meaning	Combining Form, Prefix, or Suffix
breastbone	stern/o
breathe	spir/o
breathing	-pnea
bring forth	-para
	-parous
bronchial tube (bronchus)	bronch/o
	bronchi/o
bronchiole	bronchiol/o
bunion	bunion/o
burn	caus/o
	cauter/o
bursa	burs/o
bursting forth of blood	-rrhage
	-rrhagia
calcaneus	calcane/o
calcium	calc/o
	calci/o
calculus	lith/o
calyx	cali/o
	calic/o
cancerous	carcin/o
capillary	capillar/o
carbon dioxide	capn/o
	-capnia
care for (to)	comi/o
carry	duct/o
	-ferent
	-phoria
carrying	-phoresis
cartilage	chondr/o
cast; throw	bol/o
cause	eti/o

Chart continued on following page

English—Medical Word Parts Continued

Meaning	Combining Form, Prefix, or Suffix
cecum	cec/o
cell	cyt/o
	-cyte
cells, condition of	-cytosis
cerebellum	cerebell/o
cerebrum	cerebr/o
cerumen	cerumin/o
cervix	cervic/o
change	meta-
cheek	bucc/o
chemical	chem/o
chest	pector/o
	steth/o
	thorac/o
	-thorax
child	ped/o
chin	ment/o
cholesterol	cholesterol/o
chorion	chori/o
	chorion/o
choroid layer (of the eye)	choroid/o
ciliary body (of the eye)	cycl/o
circle or cycle	cycl/o
clavicle (collar bone)	clavicul/o
clot	thromb/o
clumping	agglutin/o
clusters	staphyl/o
coagulation	coagul/o
coal dust	anthrac/o
coccyx	coccyg/o
cold	cry/o
collar bone	clavicul/o
colon	col/o (use with -ectomy, -itis, -pexy, -stomy)
colon	colon/o (use with -ic, -pathy, -scope, -scopy)

English—Medical Word Parts *Continued*

Meaning	Combining Form, Prefix, or Suffix
color	chrom/o
come together	-fusion
common bile duct	choledoch/o
complete	dia-
	tel/o
condition	-ation
	-ema
	-esis
	-ia
	-ism
	-sis
	-y
condition, abnormal	-iasis
	-osis
connect	nect/o
connective tissue	sarc/o
constant	home/o
control	-stasis, -stat
contraction	-stalsis
contraction of muscles, sudden	-spasm
coordination	tax/o
copy	-mimetic
cornea (of the eye)	corne/o
	kerat/o
cortex	cortic/o
cotton dust	byssin/o
crooked	scoli/o
crush (to)	-tripsy
curve	lord/o
cut	cis/o
	sect/o, -section
	tom/o
cut off	syncop/o
cutting, process of	-tomy

Chart continued on following page

English—Medical Word Parts *Continued*

Meaning	Combining Form, Prefix, or Suffix
cycle	cycl/o
cyst (sac of fluid)	cyst/o
dance	chore/o
dark	phe/o
darkness	scot/o
dawn-colored	eosin/o
death	leth/o
	mort/o, -mortem
	necr/o
defecation	-chezia
deficiency	-penia
deficient	hypo-
destroy	-lytic
destruction	-lysis
development	plas/o
	-plasia
	troph/o
	-trophy
diaphragm	phren/o
difficult	dys-
digestion	-pepsia
dilation	-ectasia
	-ectasis
dim	ambly/o
discharge	-rrhea
disease	nos/o
	path/o
	-pathy
distant	dist/o
	tele/o
distinct	idi/o
double	dipl/o
down	cata-
	de-

English—Medical Word Parts *Continued*

Meaning	Combining Form, Prefix, or Suffix
droop	-ptosis
drug	chem/o
	pharmac/o
	pharmaceut/o
dry	ichthy/o
	xer/o
drying	desicc/o
duct	vas/o
dull	ambly/o
duodenum	duoden/o
dura mater	dur/o
dusky	phe/o
dust	coni/o
ear	aur/o (use with -al, -icle)
	auricul/o (use with -ar)
	ot/o (use with -algia, -ic, -itis, -logy, -mycosis, -rrhea, -sclerosis, -scope, -scopy)
ear (condition of)	-otia
eardrum	myring/o (use with -ectomy, -itis, -tomy)
	tympan/o (use with -ic, -metry, -plasty)
eat	phag/o
	-phage
eating	-phagia
egg cell	o/o
	ov/o
	ovul/o
elbow	olecran/o
electricity	electr/o
elimination of wastes	-chezia

Chart continued on following page

English—Medical Word Parts *Continued*

Meaning	Combining Form, Prefix, or Suffix
embryonic	-blast
enlargement	-megaly
enzyme	-ase
epididymis	epididym/o
epiglottis	epiglott/o
equal	is/o
esophagus	esophag/o
eustachian tube	salping/o
excess	ultra-
excessive	hyper-
excision	-ectomy
expansion	-ectasia
	-ectasis
extreme	pol/o
extreme point	acr/o
extremities	acr/o
eye	ocul/o (use with -ar, -facial, -motor)
	ophthalm/o (use with -ia, -ic, -logist, -logy, -pathy, -plasty, -plegia, -scope, -scopy)
	opt/o (use with -ic, -metrist)
	optic/o (use with -al, -ian)
eyelid	blephar/o (use with -chalasis, -itis, -plasty, -plegia, -ptosis, -tomy)
	palpebr/o (use with -al)
face	faci/o
faint	syncop/o
fall	-ptosis
fallopian tube	salping/o
	-salpinx

English—Medical Word Parts *Continued*

Meaning	Combining Form, Prefix, or Suffix
false	pseudo-
far	dist/o
fascia	fasci/o
fast	tachy-
fat	adip/o (use with -ose, -osis)
	lip/o (use with -ase, -cyte, -genesis, -oid, -oma)
	steat/o (use with -oma, -rrhea)
fear	phob/o
	-phobia
feeling	esthesi/o
	-phoria
female	estr/o (use with -gen, -genic)
	gynec/o (use with -logist, -logy, -mastia)
femur	femor/o
fever	pyr/o
	pyret/o
	pyrex/o
fiber	fibr/o
fibrous connective tissue	fibros/o
fibula	fibul/o (use with -ar)
	perone/o (use with -al)
finger and toe bones	phalang/o
fingers	dactyl/o
fire	pyr/o
first	prot/o
fixation	-pexy
flat plate	-elasma
flesh	sarc/o
flow	-rrhea

Chart continued on following page

English—Medical Word Parts Continued

Meaning	Combining Form, Prefix, or Suffix
fluid collection	-oma
flushed	erythem/o
foot	pod/o
foot bones	metatars/o
forking	furc/o
form	morph/o
formation	plas/o
	-plasia
	-plasm
	-poiesis
forming	-genesis
forward	ante-, pro-, pros-
four	quadri-
front	anter/o
full of	-ose
fungus	fung/i (use with -cide, -oid, -ous, -stasis)
	myc/o (use with -logist, -logy, -osis, -tic)
gall	bil/i (use with -ary)
	chol/e (use with -lithiasis)
gallbladder	cholecyst/o
ganglion	gangli/o
	ganglion/o
gas	pneum/o
	pneumon/o
gather	-agon
genetic change	mut/a
	mutagen/o
give (to)	-dote
given (what is)	-dote
gland	aden/o

English—Medical Word Parts *Continued*

Meaning	Combining Form, Prefix, or Suffix
glans penis	balan/o
glass	silic/o
	vitre/o
globe-shaped	spher/o
glomerulus	glomerul/o
glucose	gluc/o
	glyc/o
	glycos/o
glue	coll/a
	gli/o
glycogen	glycogen/o
go (to)	-grade
good	eu-
granule(s)	granul/o
gray	glauc/o
gray matter	poli/o
green	chlor/o
groin	inguin/o
grow	-physis
growth	-plasia
gum	gingiv/o
habit	-hexia
hair	pil/o
	trich/o
half	hemi-
	semi-
hallucination	hallucin/o
hand	chir/o
hand bones	metacarp/o
hang (to)	pend/o
hard	kerat/o
	scirrh/o
hardening	-sclerosis

Chart continued on following page

English—Medical Word Parts *Continued*

Meaning	Combining Form, Prefix, or Suffix
head	cephal/o
hearing	acous/o
	audi/o
	audit/o
	-acusis
	-cusis
heart	cardi/o (use with -ac, -graphy, -logy, -logist, -megaly, -pathy, -vascular)
	coron/o (use with -ary)
heart muscle	mycardi/o
heat	cauter/o
	therm/o
heavy	pachy-
heel bone	calcane/o
hemoglobin	hemoglobin/o
hernia	-cele
	herni/o
hidden	crypt/o
hip	pelv/i
hold back	isch/o
hormone	hormon/o
	-one
horny	kerat/o
horse	equin/o
humerus	humer/o
humpback	kyph/o
hydrochloric acid	chlorhydr/o
ileum	ile/o
ilium	ili/o
immature	-blast
immature tumor (cells)	-blastoma
immune	immun/o

English—Medical Word Parts *Continued*

Meaning	Combining Form, Prefix, or Suffix
in, into, within	em-
	en-
	endo-
	in-, intra-
	ir-
in due measure	emmetr/o
in front of	pre-
incomplete	atel/o
increase in numbers (blood cells)	-cytosis
individual	idi/o
infection	seps/o
inferior to	infra-
inflammation	-itis
instrument for recording	-graph
instrument for visual examination	-scope
instrument to cut	-tome
insulin	insulin/o
internal organs	splanchn/o
	viscer/o
intestine, large	col/o
intestine, small	enter/o
iodine	iod/o
ion	ion/o
iris	ir/o
	irid/o
iron	sider/o
irregular	poikil/o
irrigation	-clysis
ischium	ischi/o
itching	prurit/o
jaw, lower	mandibul/o
	submaxill/o

Chart continued on following page

English—Medical Word Parts *Continued*

Meaning	Combining Form, Prefix, or Suffix
jaw, upper	maxill/o
joint	arthr/o
	articul/o
ketones	ket/o
	keton/o
kidney	nephr/o (use with -algia, -ectomy, -ic, -itis, -lith, -megaly, -oma, -osis, -pathy, -ptosis, -sclerosis, -stomy, -tomy)
	ren/o (use with -al, -gram, -vascular)
killing	-cidal
	-cide
knowledge	gnos/o
labor	-partum
	toc/o
	-tocia
labor (substance for)	-tocin
lack of	de-
lack of strength	-asthenia
lacrimal duct	dacry/o
	lacrim/o
lacrimal sac	dacryocyst/o
lamina	lamin/o
large	macro-
	mega-
larynx	laryng/o
lead (to)	duct/o
lens of eye	phac/o
	phak/o

English—Medical Word Parts *Continued*

Meaning	Combining Form, Prefix, or Suffix
less	de-
	mi/o
life	bi/o
	vit/o
	viv/o
ligament	ligament/o
	syndesm/o
like	phil/o
lip	cheil/o
	labi/o
lipid (fat)	lip/o
little	-ole
	-ule
liver	hepat/o
lobe	lob/o
location	top/o
loin	lumb/o
loosening	-lysis
love	phil/o
luminous	fluor/o
lung	pneum/o (use with -coccus, -coniosis, -thorax)
	pneumon/o (use with -ectomy, -ia, -ic, -itis, -lysis)
	pulmon/o (use with -ary)
lymph	lymph/o
lymph gland	lymphaden/o
lymph vessel	lymphangi/o
make (to)	-fication
male	andr/o

Chart continued on following page

English—Medical Word Parts *Continued*

Meaning	Combining Form, Prefix, or Suffix
malformed fetus	terat/o
malleolus	malleol/o
mandible	mandibul/o
	submaxill/o
many	multi-
	ple/o
	poly-
marketplace	agora-
marrow	medull/o
mass	-oma
mastoid process	mastoid/o
maxilla	maxill/o
meal	cib/o
	-prandial
measure	-meter
	metr/o
meatus	meat/o
mediastinum	mediastin/o
medulla oblongata	medull/o
meninges	mening/o
	meningi/o
menstruation; menses	men/o
metacarpals	metacarp/o
metatarsals	metatars/o
middle	medi/o
	medull/o
	meso-
middle ear	tympan/o
midwife	obstetr/o
milk	galact/o
	lact/o
mimic	-mimetic
mind	ment/o
	phren/o
	psych/o
	thymia
	-thymic

English—Medical Word Parts *Continued*

Meaning	Combining Form, Prefix, or Suffix
mixture	cras/o
monster	terat/o
more	ple/o
mouth	or/o (use with -al)
	stomat/o (use with -itis)
	-stomia
movement	cine/o
	kines/o
	kinesi/o
	-kinesia
	-kinesis
	-motor
much	poly-
mucous membrane	mucos/o
mucus	muc/o
	myx/o
muscle	muscul/o (use with -ar, -skeletal)
	my/o (use with -algia, -ectomy, -oma, -neural, -pathy, -rrhaphy, -therapy)
	myos/o (use with -in, -itis)
muscle, heart	myocardi/o
muscle, smooth (visceral)	leiomy/o
muscle, striated (skeletal)	rhabdomy/o
muscle tumor	myom/o
muzzle	phim/o
nail	onych/o
	ungu/o
narrowing	-constriction
	-stenosis

Chart continued on following page

English—Medical Word Parts *Continued*

Meaning	Combining Form, Prefix, or Suffix
nature	physi/o
navel	omphal/o
	umbilic/o
near	para-
	proxim/o
neck	cervic/o
neither	neutr/o
nerve	neur/o
nerve root	radicul/o
nest	nid/o
new	neo-
network	reticul/o
network of nerves	plex/o
neutral	neutr/o
neutrophil	neutr/o
night	noct/i
	nyct/o
nipple	thel/o
nipple-like	papill/o
nitrogen	azot/o
nitrogen compound	-amine
no, not	a-
	an-
none	nulli-
normal	eu-
nose	nas/o (use with -al)
	rhin/o (use with -itis, -rrhea, -plasty)
nourishment	troph/o
	-trophy
nucleus	kary/o
	nucle/o
nucleus (collection of nerve cells in the brain)	kern-
numbness	narc/o

English—Medical Word Parts *Continued*

Meaning	Combining Form, Prefix, or Suffix
obscure	-opaque
obsessive preoccupation	-mania
off	apo-
old age	ger/o
	presby/o
olecranon (elbow)	olecran/o
on	epi-
one	mon/o
	mono-
	uni-
one's own	aut/o
	auto-
one who	-er
	-or
opening	-tresia
opening (new)	-stomy
opposite	contra-
optic disc (disk)	papill/o
orange-yellow	cirrh/o
order	norm/o
	tax/o
organs, internal	viscer/o
ossicle	ossicul/o
other	all/o
other than	par-
out, outside	ec-
	ex-
	exo-
	extra-
outer region	cortic/o
ovary	oophor/o (use with -itis, -ectomy, -pexy)
	ovari/o (use with -an)
oxygen	ox/o
	-oxia

Chart continued on following page

English—Medical Word Parts *Continued*

Meaning	Combining Form, Prefix, or Suffix
pain	-algia
	-dynia
	odyn/o
pain, excessive	-agra
pain, sensitivity to	-algesia
	algesi/o
painful	dys-
palate	palat/o
palsy	-plegia
	-plegic
pancreas	pancreat/o
paralysis	-plegia
	-plegic
paralysis, slight	-paresis
patella	patell/a (use with -pexy)
	patell/o (use with -ar, -ectomy, -femoral)
pelvic bone, pelvis	pelv/i
	pelv/o
penis	balan/o
	phall/o
people	dem/o
perineum	perine/o
peritoneum	peritone/o
pertaining to	-ac (cardiac)
	-al (inguinal)
	-an (ovarian)
	-ar (palmar)
	-ary (papillary)
	-eal (pharyngeal)
	-iac (hypochondriac)
	-ic (nucleic)
	-ical (neurological)
	-ine (equine)
	-ior (superior)

English—Medical Word Parts *Continued*

Meaning	Combining Form, Prefix, or Suffix
pertaining to, *continued*	-ose (adipose)
	-ous (mucous)
	-tic (necrotic)
phalanges	phalang/o
pharynx (throat)	pharyng/o
phrase	-lexia
physician	iatr/o
pineal gland	pineal/o
pituitary gland	hypophys/o
	pituit/o
	pituitar/o
place	-stasis
	the/o
	top/o
plant	phyt/o
	-phyte
plaque	ather/o
	-plakia
pleura	pleur/o
pleural cavity	-thorax
plexus	plex/o
poison	tox/o
	toxic/o
pole	styl/o
polyp	polyp/o
pons	pont/o
pores (condition of)	-porosis
position	top/o
potassium	kal/i
pour	chym/o
	-fusion
pregnancy	-cyesis
	gest/o
	gester/o

Chart continued on following page

English—Medical Word Parts *Continued*

Meaning	Combining Form, Prefix, or Suffix
pregnancy, *continued*	gravid/o
	-gravida
pressure	bar/o
	-tension
process	-ation
	-ion
	-ism
	-y
produced by or in	-genic
producing	-gen
	-genesis
prolapse	-ptosis
prostate gland	prostat/o
protection	immun/o
	-phylaxis
protein	-globin
	-globulin
	prote/o
pubis	pub/o
pulse	sphygm/o
	-sphyxia
puncture to remove fluid	-centesis
pupil	cor/o
	core/o
	pupill/o
pus	py/o, purul/o
put	the/o
put in place	-pexy
pyloric sphincter, pylorus	pylor/o
radioactivity	radi/o
radius (lower arm bone)	radi/o
rapid	oxy-

English—Medical Word Parts *Continued*

Meaning	Combining Form, Prefix, or Suffix
rash	exanthemat/o
rays	radi/o
record	-gram
recording, process of	-graphy
rectum	rect/o
recurring	cycl/o
red	erythr/o
redness	erythem/o
	erythemat/o
reduce	-lytic
relaxation	-chalasia, -chalasis
removal	-apheresis
	-ectomy
	-pheresis
renal pelvis	pyel/o
repair	-plasty
resembling	-form
	-oid
retina	retin/o
rib	cost/o
roll (to)	vol/o
rosy	eosin/o
round	spher/o
rule	norm/o
run	-drome
rupture	-rrhexis
sac, small	alveol/o
	follicul/o
sac of fluid	cyst/o
sacrum	sacr/o
safe	immun/o
sag (to)	-ptosis
saliva	sial/o

Chart continued on following page

English—Medical Word Parts *Continued*

Meaning	Combining Form, Prefix, or Suffix
salivary gland	sialaden/o
same	ipsi-
	is/o
sameness	home/o
scaly	ichthy/o
scanty	olig/o
sclera	scler/o
scrotum	scrot/o
sea	thalass/o
sebum	seb/o
	sebace/o
	steat/o
secrete	crin/o
	-crine
seed	gon/o
	semin/i
seizure	-lepsy
seize (to); take hold of	-leptic
self	aut/o
	auto-
semen	semin/i
seminal vesicle	vesicul/o
send (to)	-mission
sensation (nervous)	-esthesia
separate	-crine
	-lytic
separation	-lysis
set (to)	-stitial
severe	acu/o
sex glands	gonad/o
sexual intercourse	-pareunia
shape	-form
	morph/o
sharp	acu/o
	oxy-
sheath	thec/o

English—Medical Word Parts *Continued*

Meaning	Combining Form, Prefix, or Suffix
sodium	natr/o
soft	medull/o
softening	-malacia
sole (of the foot)	plant/o
solution	-sol
sound	echo-
	-phon/o
	-phonia
	son/o
spark	scint/i
specialist	-ist
speech	phas/o
	-phasia
sperm cells (spermatozoa)	sperm/o
	spermat/o
spinal column	rachi/o
spinal cord	myel/o
spinal column (spine)	spin/o
	rachi/o
	vertebr/o
spiny	acanth/o
spitting	-ptysis
spleen	splen/o
split	-fida
	schiz/o
split (to)	-schisis
stake (pole)	styl/o
stapes	staped/o
starch	amyl/o
state of	-sis
steal	klept/o
sternum	stern/o
steroid	ster/o
sticking together	agglutin/o
stiff	ankyl/o
stimulate	-tropin

English—Medical Word Parts *Continued*

Meaning	Combining Form, Prefix, or Suffix
shield	thyr/o
shin bone	tibi/o
shine	-lucent
short	brachy-
shoulder	om/o
side	later/o
sieve	ethm/o
sigmoid colon	sigmoid/o
single	mon/o
sinus	sinus/o
skin	cutane/o (use with -ous)
	derm/o (use with -al)
	-derma (use with erythr/o, leuk/o)
	dermat/o (use with -itis, -logist, -logy, -osis)
	epitheli/o (use with -al, -lysis, -oid, -oma, -um)
skull	crani/o
sleep	hypn/o
	somn/o
	-somnia
sleep (deep)	comat/o
slender	lept/o
slide (to)	-lapse
	lux/o
slipping	-listhesis
slow	brady-
small	-icle
	micro-
	-ole
	-ule
small intestine	enter/o
smaller	mi/o
smell	-osmia

Chart continued on following page

English—Medical Word Parts *Continued*

Meaning	Combining Form, Prefix, or Suffix
stomach	gastr/o
stone	lith/o
stop	-suppression
stopping	-stasis
	-static
straight	orth/o
stranger	xen/o
strength	-sthenia
stretch	tone/o
stretching	-ectasia
	-ectasis
stricture	-stenosis
structure	-ium
	-um, -us
structure, solid	ster/o
study of	log/o-
	-logy
stupor	narc/o
substance	-in
	-ine
substance that forms	-poietin
sudden	acu/o
	oxysm/o
sugar	gluc/o
	glyc/o
	glycos/o
	-ose
surgical repair	-plasty
surrounding	peri-
suture (to)	-rrhaphy
swallow	phag/o
swallowing	-phagia
swayback	lord/o
sweat	diaphor/o (use with -esis)
	hidr/o (use with -osis)

Chart continued on following page

English—Medical Word Parts *Continued*

Meaning	Combining Form, Prefix, or Suffix
swift	oxy-
sword	xiph/o
synovia (fluid)	synov/o
synovial membrane	synov/o
tail	caud/o
tailbone	coccyg/o
tear	dacry/o (use with -genic, -rrhea)
	lacrim/o (use with -al, -ation)
tear (to cut)	-spadia
tear gland	dacryoaden/o
tear sac	dacryocyst/o
temperament	cras/o
tendon	ten/o
	tend/o
	tendin/o
tension	ton/o
testis	orch/o (use with -itis)
	orchi/o (use with -algia, -dynia, -ectomy, -pathy, -pexy, -tomy)
	orchid/o (use with -ectomy, -pexy, -plasty, -ptosis, -tomy)
	test/o (use with -sterone)
thick	pachy-
thigh bone	femor/o
thin	lept/o
thing	-um
	-us
thirst	dips/o
thorny	acanth/o
three	tri-
throat	pharyng/o

English—Medical Word Parts *Continued*

Meaning	Combining Form, Prefix, or Suffix
through	dia-
	per-
	trans-
throw (to)	bol/o
thymus gland	thym/o
thyroid gland	thyr/o
	thyroid/o
tibia	tibi/o
tie	nect/o
tie together	-desis
tightening	-stenosis
time	chron/o
tissue	hist/o
	histi/o
	-ium
	-um
toes	dactyl/o
together	con-
	sym-
	syn-
tongue	gloss/o (use with -al, -dynia, -plasty, -plegia, -rrhaphy, -spasm, -tomy)
	lingu/o (use with -al)
tonsil	tonsill/o
tooth	dent/i
	odont/o
top	acr/o
toward	ad-
	af-
trachea	trache/o
transmission	-phoresis
treatment	iatr/o
	therapeut/o
	-therapy
trigone	trigon/o

Chart continued on following page

English—Medical Word Parts *Continued*

Meaning	Combining Form, Prefix, or Suffix
tube	syring/o
tumor	-oma
	onc/o
turn	-tropia
	-verse
	-version
turning	-tropic
twisted chains	strept/o
two	bi-
tympanic membrane	myring/o
	tympan/o
ulcer	aphth/o
ulna	uln/o
umbilicus, navel	omphal/o (use with -cele, -ectomy, -rrhagia, -rrhexis)
	umbilic/o (use with -al)
unchanging	home/o
under	hypo-
unequal	anis/o
unknown	idi/o
up	ana-
upon	epi-
urea	azot/o
ureter	ureter/o
urethra	urethr/o
urinary bladder	cyst/o (use with cele, -ectomy, -itis, -pexy, -plasty, -plegia, -scope, -scopy, -stomy, -tomy)
	vesic/o (use with -al)
urinary tract	ur/o
urination	-uria

English—Medical Word Parts *Continued*

Meaning	Combining Form, Prefix, or Suffix
urine	ur/o
	-uria
	urin/o
uterus	hyster/o (use with -ectomy, -graphy, -gram, -tomy)
	metr/o (use with -rrhagia, -rrhea, -rrhexis)
	metri/o (use with -osis)
	uter/o (use with –ine)
uvea	uve/o
uvula	uvul/o (use with -ar, -itis, -ptosis)
	staphyl/o (use with -ectomy, -plasty, -tomy)
vagina	colp/o (use with -pexy, -plasty, -scope, -scopy, -tomy)
	vagin/o (use with -al, -itis)
vagus nerve	vag/o
valve	valv/o
	valvul/o
varicose veins	varic/o
varied	poikil/o
vas deferens	vas/o
vein	phleb/o (use with -ectomy, -itis, -tomy)
	ven/o (use with -ous, -gram)
	ven/i (use with -puncture)
vein, small	venul/o

Chart continued on following page

English—Medical Word Parts *Continued*

Meaning	Combining Form, Prefix, or Suffix
venereal	vener/o
ventricle	ventricul/o
vertebra	rachi/o (use with -itis, -tomy)
	spondyl/o (use with -itis, -listhesis, -osis, -pathy)
	vertebr/o (use with -al)
vessel	angi/o (use with -ectomy, -genesis, -gram, -graphy, -oma, -plasty, -spasm)
	vas/o (use with -constriction, -dilation, -motor)
	vascul/o (use with -ar, -itis)
view of	-opsy
viscera	splanchn/o
vision	-opia
	-opsia
	opt/o
	optic/o
visual examination	-scopy
vitreous body	vitr/o
voice	phon/o
	-phonia
voice box	laryng/o
vomiting	-emesis
vulva	episi/o (use with -tomy)
	vulv/o (use with -ar)
wander	ion/o
washing	-clysis
wasting away	-phthisis
water	aque/o
	hydr/o

English—Medical Word Parts *Continued*

Meaning	Combining Form, Prefix, or Suffix
watery flow	rheumat/o
wedge	sphen/o
weight	bar/o
white	alb/o
	albin/o
	leuk/o
wide	mydr/o
widening	-dilation
	-ectasia
	-ectasis
	-eurysm
windpipe	trache/o
with	con-
	sym-
	syn-
within	en-
	endo-
	intra-
woman	gynec/o
womb	hyster/o
	metr/o
	metri/o
	uter/o
word	-lexia
work	erg/o
wrinkle	rhytid/o
wrist bone	carp/o
x-rays	radi/o
yellow	lute/o
	jaund/o
	xanth/o

Abbreviations*

Many of these abbreviations may appear with or without periods and with either a capital or a lowercase first letter.

@	at
$\bar{a}$	before
A, B, AB, O	blood types; may have subscript numbers
A2 or A_2	aortic valve closure (heart sound)
AAA	abdominal aortic aneurysm
AAL	anterior axillary line
AB/ab	abortion
Ab	antibody
ABCD	asymetry, border, color, diameter (description of skin cancerous lesions)
abd	abdomen; abduction
ABG	arterial blood gas
a.c.	before meals *(ante cibum)*
ACE	angiotensin-converting enzyme (ACE inhibitors are used to treat hypertension)
ACh	acetylcholine (neurotransmitter)
ACL	anterior cruciate ligament (of knee)
ACS	acute coronary syndromes
ACTH	adrenocorticotropic hormone (secreted by the anterior pituitary gland)
AD	right ear *(auris dextra);* Alzheimer disease
ADD	attention deficit disorder
add	adduction
ADH	antidiuretic hormone; vasopressin (secreted by the posterior pituitary gland)

Chart continued on following page

*From Chabner D-E: The Language of Medicine, 7th ed. Philadelphia, WB Saunders, 2004.

Abbreviations *Continued*

ADHD	attention-deficit hyperactivity disorder
ADL	activity of daily living
ADT	admission, discharge, transfer
ad lib	as desired
AF	atrial fibrillation
AFB	acid-fast bacillus (bacilli); TB organism
AFO	ankle foot orthosis (device for stabilization)
AFP	alpha-fetoprotein
Ag	silver
AHF	antihemophilic factor (coagulation factor XIII or IX)
AIDS	acquired immunodeficiency syndrome
AIHA	autoimmune hemolytic anemia
AKA	above-knee amputation
alb	albumin (protein)
alk phos	alkaline phosphatase (elevated in liver disease)
ALL	acute lymphocytic leukemia
ALS	amyotrophic lateral sclerosis (Lou Gehrig disease)
ALT	alanine aminotransferase (elevated in liver and heart disease); formerly SGPT
a.m. or AM	in the morning or before noon
AMA	against medical advice; American Medical Association
Amb	ambulate, ambulatory (walking)
AML	acute myelocytic (myelogenous) leukemia
ANC	absolute neutrophil count
AP or A/P	anteroposterior
A&P	auscultation and percussion
APC	acetylsalicylic acid (aspirin), phenacetin, and caffeine
aq.	water *(aqua);* aqueous
ARDS	adult respiratory distress syndrome
AROM	active range of motion
AS	left ear *(auris sinistra);* aortic stenosis
ASA	acetylsalicylic acid (aspirin)
ASD	atrial septal defect

Abbreviations *Continued*

ASHD	arteriosclerotic heart disease
AST	aspartate aminotransferase (elevated in liver and heart disease); formerly SGOT
AU	each ear, both ears *(auris uterque)*
Au	gold
AV	arteriovenous; atrioventricular
AVM	arteriovenous malformation
AVR	aortic valve replacement
A&W	alive and well
Ba	barium
BAL	bronchioalveolar lavage
bands	banded neutrophils
baso	basophils
BBB	bundle branch block
BC	bone conduction
B cells	lymphocytes produced in the bone marrow
BE	barium enema
b.i.d.	twice a day *(bis in die)*
BKA	below-knee amputation
BM	bowel movement
BMR	basal metabolic rate
BMT	bone marrow transplant
BP or B/P	blood pressure
BPH	benign prostatic hyperplasia (hypertrophy)
BRBPR	bright red blood per rectum; hematochezia
BSE	breast self examination
BSO	bilateral salpingo-oophorectomy
BSP	bromsulphalein (dye used in liver function test; its retention is indicative of liver damage or disease)
BT	bleeding time
BUN	blood urea nitrogen
Bx, bx	biopsy

Chart continued on following page

Abbreviations *Continued*

C	carbon; calorie
°C	Celsius, centigrade (temperature scale)
c̄	with *(cum)*
C1, C2	first, second cervical vertebra
CA	cancer; carcinoma; cardiac arrest; chronological age
Ca	calcium
CABG	coronary artery bypass graft
CAD	coronary artery disease
CAO	chronic airway obstruction
CAPD	continuous ambulatory peritoneal dialysis
cap	capsule
Cath	catheter; catheterization
CAT	computerized axial tomography
CBC	complete blood cell count
CC	chief complaint
cc	cubic centimeter (same as ml; 1/1000 liter)
CCU	coronary care unit; critical care unit
CDC	Centers for Disease Control and Prevention
CDH	congenital dislocated hip
CEA	carcinoembryonic antigen
cf.	compare
CF	cystic fibrosis
cGy	centigray (one hundredth of a gray; a rad)
CHD	coronary heart disease; chronic heart disease
chemo	chemotherapy
CHF	congestive heart failure
chol	cholesterol
chr	chronic
μCi	microcurie
CIN	cervical intraepithelial neoplasia
CIS	carcinoma *in situ*
CK	creatine kinase
Cl	chlorine

Abbreviations *Continued*

CLD	chronic liver disease
CLL	chronic lymphocytic leukemia
cm	centimeter (1/100 meter)
CMA	certified medical assistant
CMG	cystometrogram
CML	chronic myelogenous leukemia
CMV	cytomegalovirus
CNS	central nervous sysem
Co	cobalt
c/o	complains of
CO₂	carbon dioxide
COD	condition on discharge
COPD	chronic obstructive pulmonary disease
CP	cerebral palsy; chest pain
CPA	costophrenic angle
CPAP	continuous positive airway pressure
CPD	cephalopelvic disproportion
CPK	creatine phosphokinase
CPR	cardiopulmonary resuscitation
CR	complete response; cardiorespiratory
CRF	chronic renal failure
C-section	cesarean section
C&S	culture and sensitivity
CSF	cerebrospinal fluid; colony-stimulating factor
C-spine	cervical spine films
ct.	count
CTA	clear to auscultation
CTS	carpal tunnel syndrome
CT scan	computed tomography (x-ray images in a cross-sectional view)
CT	chemotherapy
Cu	copper
CVA	cerebrovascular accident; costovertebral angle
CVP	central venous pressure
CVS	cardiovascular system; chorionic villus sampling

Chart continued on following page

Abbreviations *Continued*

c/w	compare with; consistent with
CX (CXR)	chest x- ray
Cx	cervix
cysto	cystoscopy

D/C	discontinue; discharge
D&C	dilatation (dilation) and curettage
DCIS	ductal carcinoma *in situ*
DD	discharge diagnosis
Decub.	decubitus (lying down)
Derm.	dermatology
DES	diethylstilbestrol; diffuse esophageal spasm
DI	diabetes insipidus; diagnostic imaging
DIC	disseminated intravascular coagulation
DICOM	digital image communication in medicine
diff.	differential count (white blood cells)
DIG	digoxin; digitalis
dL, dl	deciliter (1/10 liter)
DLco	diffusion capacity of the lung for carbon monoxide
DLE	discoid lupus erythematosus
DM	diabetes mellitus
DNA	deoxyribonucleic acid
DNR	do not resuscitate
D.O.	Doctor of Osteopathy
DOA	dead on arrival
DOB	date of birth
DOE	dyspnea on exertion
DPI	dry powder inhaler
DPT	diphtheria, pertussis, tetanus (vaccine)
DRE	digital rectal exam
DRG	diagnosis-related group
DSA	digital subtraction angiography
DSM	Diagnostic and Statistical Manual of Mental Disorders
DT	delirium tremens (caused by alcohol withdrawal)

Abbreviations *Continued*

DTR	deep tendon reflexes
DUB	dysfunctional uterine bleeding
DVT	deep venous thrombosis
D/W	dextrose and water
Dx	diagnosis
EBV	Epstein-Barr virus
ECC	endocervical curettage; extracorporeal circulation
ECF	extended-care facility
ECG	electrocardiogram
ECHO	echocardiography
ECMO	extracorporeal membrane oxygenation
ECT	electroconvulsive therapy
ED	emergency department
EDC	estimated date of confinement
EEG	electroencephalogram
EENT	eyes, ears, nose, and throat
EGD	esophagogastroduodenoscopy
EKG	electrocardiogram
ELISA	enzyme-linked immunosorbent assay (AIDS test)
EM	electron microscope
EMB	endometrial biopsy
EMG	electromyogram
EMT	emergency medical technician
ENT	ear, nose, and throat
EOM	extraocular movement; extraocular muscles
eos.	eosinophil (type of white blood cell)
EPO	erythropoietin
ER	emergency room; estrogen receptor
ERCP	endoscopic retrograde cholangiopancreatography
ERT	estrogen replacement therapy
ESR	erythrocyte sedimentation rate
ESRD	end-stage renal disease
ESWL	extracorporeal shock wave lithotripsy

Chart continued on following page

Abbreviations *Continued*

ETOH	ethyl alcohol
ETT	exercise tolerance test
F or °F	Fahrenheit
FACP	Fellow, American College of Physicians
FACS	Fellow, American College of Surgeons
FB	fingerbreadth; foreign body
FBS	fasting blood sugar
FDA	Food and Drug Administration
Fe	iron
FEF	forced expiratory flow
FEV₁	forced expiratory volume
FH	family history
FHR	fetal heart rate
FROM	full range of movement/motion
FSH	follicle-stimulating hormone
F/u	follow-up
5-FU	5-fluorouracil (used in cancer chemotherapy)
FUO	fever of undetermined origin
Fx	fracture
μg	microgram (one-millionth of a gram)
G	gravida (pregnant)
g, gm	gram
Ga	gallium
g/dL	gram per deciliter
GABA	gamma-aminobutyric acid (neurotransmitter)
GB	gallbladder
GBS	gallbladder series (x-rays)
GC	gonorrhea
G-CSF	granulocyte colony-stimulating factor
GERD	gastroesophageal reflux disease
GFR	glomerular filtration rate
GH	growth hormone

Abbreviations *Continued*

GI	gastrointestinal
G$_6$PD	glucose-6-phosphate dehydrogenase (enzyme missing in inherited red blood cell disorder)
GP	general practitioner
GM-CSF	granulocyte macrophage colony-stimulating factor
Grav. 1, 2, 3	first, second, third pregnancy
GTT	glucose tolerance test
gtt	drop *(gutta)*, drops *(guttae)*
GU	genitourinary
Gy	gray (unit of radiation and equal to 100 rad)
GYN or **gyn**	gynecology
H	hydrogen
h., hr	hour
H2 blocker	H2 (histamine) receptor antagonist (inhibitor of gastric acid secretion)
HAART	highly active antiretroviral therapy (for AIDS)
Hb; hgb	hemoglobin
HbA1C	glycosylated hemoglobin test (for diabetes)
HBV	hepatitis B virus
HCG **(hCG)**	human chorionic gonadotropin
HCl	hydrochloric acid
HCO$_3$	bicarbonate
Hct (HCT)	hematocrit
HCV	hepatitis C virus
HCVD	hypertensive cardiovascular disease
HD	hemodialysis (artificial kidney machine)
HDL	high-density lipoprotein
He	helium
HEENT	head, eyes, ears, nose, and throat

Chart continued on following page

Abbreviations *Continued*

Hg	mercury
H&H	hematocrit and hemoglobin
HIPAA	Health Insurance Portability and Accountability Act (of 1996)
HIV	human immunodeficiency virus
HLA	histocompatibility locus antigen (identifies cells as "self")
HNP	herniated nucleus pulposus
h/o	history of
H_2O	water
H&P	history and physical
HPF; hpf	high-power field (microscope)
HPI	history of present illness
HPV	human papillomavirus
HRT	hormone replacement therapy
h.s.	at bedtime *(hora somni)*
HSG	hysterosalpingography
HSV	herpes simplex virus
ht	height
HTN	hypertension (high blood pressure)
Hx	history
I	iodine
^{131}I	radioactive isotope of iodine
IBD	inflammatory bowel disease
ICD	implantable cardioverter/defibrillator
ICP	intracranial pressure
ICSH	interstitial cell-stimulating hormone
ICU	intensive care unit
I&D	incision and drainage
ID	infectious disease
IgA, IgD, IgE, IgG, IgM	immunoglobulins
IHD	ischemic heart disease
IHSS	idiopathic hypertrophic subaortic stenosis
IL1-15	interleukins

Abbreviations *Continued*

IM	intramuscular; infectious mononucleosis
IMV	intermittent mandatory ventilation
inf.	infusion; inferior
INH	isoniazid (drug used to treat tuberculosis)
inj.	injection
I&O	intake and output (measurement of patient's fluids)
IOL	intraocular lens (implant)
IOP	intraocular pressure
IPPB	intermittent positive pressure breathing
I.Q.	intelligence quotient
ITP	idiopathic thrombocytopenic pupura
IUD	intrauterine device
IUP	intrauterine pregnancy
IV or **I.V.**	intravenous (injection)
IVP	intravenous pyelogram
K	potassium
kg	kilogram (1000 grams)
KJ	knee jerk
KS	Kaposi sarcoma
KUB	kidney, ureter, and bladder (x-ray exam)
μl	microliter (one-millionth of a liter)
L, l	liter; left; lower
L1, L2	first, second lumbar vertebra
LA	left atrium
LAD	left anterior descending (coronary artery)
lat	lateral
LB	large bowel
LBBB	left bundle branch block (heart block)
LD	lethal dose
LDH	lactate dehydrogenase

Chart continued on following page

Abbreviations *Continued*

LDL	low-density lipoprotein (high levels associated with heart disease)
L-dopa	levodopa (used to treat Parkinson disease)
L.E.	lupus erythematosus
LEEP	loop electrocautery excision procedure
LES	lower esophageal sphincter
LFT	liver function test
LH	luteinizing hormone
LLL	left lower lobe (lung)
LLQ	left lower quadrant (abdomen)
LMP	last menstrual period
LMWP	low–molecular-weight heparin
LOC	loss of consciousness
LOS	length of stay
LP	lumbar puncture
lpf	low-power field (microscope)
LPN	licensed practical nurse
LS	lumbosacral spine
LSD	lysergic acid diethylamide
LSK	liver, spleen, and kidneys
LTB	laryngotracheal bronchitis (croup)
LTC	long-term care
LTH	luteotropic hormone (prolactin)
LUL	left upper lobe (lung)
LUQ	left upper quadrant (abdomen)
LV	left ventricle
LVAD	left ventricular assist device
L&W	living and well
lymphs	lymphocytes
lytes	electrolytes
MA	mental age
MAC	monitored anesthesia care
MAI	*Mycobacterium avium intracellulare*
MAOI	monoamine oxidase inhibitor (antidepressant drug)
MBD	minimal brain dysfunction

Abbreviations *Continued*

mcg	microgram
MCH	mean corpuscular hemoglobin (average amount in each red blood cell)
MCHC	mean corpuscular hemoglobin concentration (average concentration in a single red cell)
mCi	millicurie
μCi	microcurie
MCP	metacarpophalangeal joint
MCV	mean corpuscular volume (average size of a single red blood cell)
M.D.	Doctor of Medicine
MDI	metered-dose inhaler
MDR	minimum daily requirement
MED	minimum effective dose
mEq	milliequivalent
mEq/L	milliequivalent per liter (measurement of the concentration of a solution)
mets	metastases
MG	myasthenia gravis
Mg	magnesium
mg	milligram (1/1000 gram)
mg/cc	milligram per cubic centimeter
mg/dl	milligram per deciliter
μg	microgram (one-millionth of a gram)
MH	marital history; mental health
MI	myocardial infarction; mitral insufficiency
mL, ml	milliliter (1/1000 liter)
mm	millimeter (1/1000 meter; 0.039 inch)
mm Hg	millimeters of mercury
MMPI	Minnesota Multiphasic Personality Inventory
MMR	measles-mumps-rubella (vaccine)
MMT	manual muscle testing
mμ	millimicron (1/1000 micron; a micron is 10^{-3} mm)
μm	micrometer (one-millionth of a meter)
MOAB	monoclonal antibody

Chart continued on following page

Abbreviations *Continued*

monos	monocytes (white blood cells)
MR	mitral regurgitation
MRA	magnetic resonance angiogram
MRI	magnetic resonance imaging
mRNA	messenger RNA
MS	multiple sclerosis; mitral stenosis
MSL	midsternal line
MTX	methotrexate
MUGA	multiple-gated acquisition scan (of heart)
multip	multipara; multiparous
MVP	mitral valve prolapse
N	nitrogen
NA	not applicable
Na	sodium
NB	newborn
NBS	normal bowel or breath sounds
ND	normal delivery; normal development
NED	no evidence of disease
neg.	negative
NG tube	nasogastric tube
NHL	non-Hodgkin lymphoma
NICU	neonatal intensive care unit
NKA	no known allergies
NK cells	natural killer cells
NKDA	no known drug allergies
n.p.o.	nothing by mouth *(non per os)*
NSAID	nonsteroidal anti-inflammatory drug
NSR	normal sinus rhythm (of heart)
NTP	normal temperature and pressure
O or O$_2$	oxygen
OA	osteoarthritis
OB/GYN	obstetrics and gynecology
OCPs	oral contraceptive pills
O.D.	Doctor of Optometry
OD	right eye *(oculus dexter);* overdose

Abbreviations *Continued*

OR	operating room
ORIF	open reduction internal fixation
ORTH; **Ortho.**	orthopedics
OS	left eye *(oculus sinister)*
os	opening; bone
O.T.	occupational therapy
OU	each eye *(oculus uterque)*
oz.	ounce
P	phosphorus; posterior; pressure; pulse; pupil
p̄	after
P2 or P₂	pulmonary valve closure (heart sound)
PA	pulmonary artery; posteroanterior; physician's assistant
P/A	posteroanterior
P&A	percussion and auscultation
PAC	premature atrial contraction
PACS	picture archival communications system
PaCO₂, pCO₂	partial pressure of carbon dioxide in blood
palp.	palpable; palpation
PALS	pediatric advanced life support
PaO₂, pO₂	partial pressure of oxygen in blood
Pap smear	Papanicolaou smear (cells from cervix and vagina)
Para 1, 2, 3	unipara, bipara, tripara (number of viable births)
p.c.	after meals *(post cibum)*
PCA	patient-controlled anesthesia
PCI	percutaneous coronary interventions
PCP	*Pneumocystis carinii* pneumonia; phencyclidine (hallucinogen)
PCR	polymerase chain reaction (process allows making copies of genes)
PD	peritoneal dialysis

Chart continued on following page

Abbreviations *Continued*

PDA	patent ductus arteriosus
PDR	Physicians' Desk Reference
PE	physical examination; pulmonary embolism
PEEP	positive end-expiratory pressure
PEG	percutaneous endoscopic gastrostomy (a feeding tube)
PEJ	percutaneous endoscopic jejunostomy (a feeding tube)
per os	by mouth
PERRLA	pupils equal, round, react to light and accommodation
PET	positron emission tomography
PE tube	ventilating tube for eardrum
PFT	pulmonary function test
PG	prostaglandin
PH	past history
pH	hydrogen ion concentration (alkalinity and acidity measurement)
PI	present illness
PID	pelvic inflammatory disease
PIP	proximal interphalangeal joint
PKU	phenylketonuria
p.m. or PM	afternoon (post meridian)
PMH	past medical history
PMN	polymorphonuclear leukocyte
PMS	premenstrual syndrome
PND	paroxysmal nocturnal dyspnea
p/o	postoperative
p.o.	by mouth *(per os)*
poly	polymorphonuclear leukocyte
postop	postoperative (after surgery)
PPBS	postprandial blood sugar
PPD	purified protein derivative (test for tuberculosis)
preop	preoperative
prep	prepare for
PR	partial response
primip	primipara
PRL	prolactin

Abbreviations *Continued*

p.r.n.	as required *(pro re nata)*
procto	proctoscopy
prot.	protocol
Pro. time	prothrombin time (test of blood clotting)
PSA	prostate-specific antigen
PT	prothrombin time; physical therapy
PTA	prior to admission (to hospital)
PTC	percutaneous transhepatic cholangiography
PTCA	percutaneous transluminal coronary angioplasty
PTH	parathyroid hormone
PTHC	percutaneous transhepatic cholangiography
PTSD	post-traumatic stress disorder
PTT	partial thromboplastin time (test of blood clotting)
PU	pregnancy urine
PUVA therapy	psoralen ultraviolet A (treatment for psoriasis)
PVC	premature ventricular contraction
PVD	peripheral vascular disease
PWB	partial weight bearing
Px	prognosis

q	every *(quaque)*
qAM	every morning
q.d.	every day *(quaque die)*
q.h.	every hour *(quaque hora)*
q.2h.	every 2 hours
q.i.d.	four times daily *(quater in die)*
qns	quantity not sufficient
qPM	every evening
QRS	wave complex in an electrocardiographic study
q.s.	as much as suffices *(quantum sufficit)*
qt	quart

Chart continued on following page

Abbreviations *Continued*

R	respiration; right
RA	rheumatoid arthritis; right atrium
Ra	radium
rad	radiation absorbed dose
RBBB	right bundle branch block
RBC, rbc	red blood cell (corpuscle); red blood count
R.D.D.A.	recommended daily dietary allowance
RDS	respiratory distress syndrome
REM	rapid eye movement
RF	rheumatoid factor
Rh (factor)	rhesus (monkey) factor in blood
RIA	radioimmunoassay (minute quantities are measured)
RLL	right lower lobe (lung)
RLQ	right lower quadrant (abdomen)
RML	right middle lobe (lung)
RNA	ribonucleic acid
R/O	rule out
ROM	range of motion
ROS	review of systems
RRR	regular rate and rhythm (of the heart)
RT	right; radiation therapy
RUL	right upper lobe (lung)
RUQ	right upper quadrant (abdomen)
RV	right ventricle
Rx	treatment; therapy; prescription
s̄	without *(sine)*
S1, S2	first, second sacral vertebra
S-A node	sinoatrial node (pacemaker of heart)
SAD	seasonal affective disorder
SARS	severe acute respiratory syndrome
SBE	subacute bacterial endocarditis
SBFT	small bowel follow-through (x-rays of small intestine)
SC	subcutaneous
sed. rate	sedimentation rate (rate of erythrocyte sedimentation)

Abbreviations *Continued*

segs	segmented neutrophils; polys
SERM	selective estrogen receptor modifier
SGOT (AST)	serum glutamic-oxaloacetic transaminase
SGPT (ALT)	serum glutamic-pyruvic transaminase
SIADH	syndrome of inappropriate antidiuretic hormone
SIDS	sudden infant death syndrome
sig.	let it be labeled
SL	sublingual
SLE	systemic lupus erythematosus
SMAC	automated analytical device for testing blood
SMA 12	twelve blood chemistries
SOAP	subjective, objective, assessment, and plan (used for patient notes)
SOB	shortness of breath
s.o.s.	if necessary *(si opus sit)*
S/P	status post (previous disease condition)
SPECT	single-photon emission computed tomography
sp. gr.	specific gravity
s/s	signs and symptoms
SSCP	substernal chest pain
SSRI	selective serotonin reuptake inhibitor (antidepressant)
Staph.	staphylococci (berry-shaped bacteria in clusters)
stat.	immediately *(statim)*
STH	somatotropin (growth hormone)
Strep.	streptococci (berry-shaped bacteria in twisted chains)
subcut	subcutaneous
SVC	superior vena cava
SVD	spontaneous vaginal delivery
Sx	symptoms
Sz	seizure

Chart continued on following page

Abbreviations *Continued*

T	temperature; time
T tube	tube placed in biliary tract for drainage
T1, T2	first, second thoracic vertebra
T_3	triiodothyronine test
T_4	thyroxine test
TA	therapeutic abortion
T&A	tonsillectomy and adenoidectomy
TAB	therapeutic abortion
TAH	total abdominal hysterectomy
TAT	Thematic Apperception Test
TB	tuberculosis
Tc	technetium
T cells	lymphocytes produced in the thymus gland
T tube	tube placed in biliary tract for drainage
TEE	transesophageal echocardiogram
TENS	transcutaneous electrical nerve stimulation
TFT	thyroid function test
TIA	transient ischemic attack
t.i.d.	three times daily *(ter in die)*
TLC	total lung capacity
TM	tympanic membrane
TMJ	temporomandibular joint
TNM	tumor, nodes, and metastases
tPA	tissue plasminogen activator
TPN	total parenteral nutrition
TPR	temperature, pulse, and respiration
TRUS	transrectal ultrasound
TSH	thyroid-stimulating hormone
TSS	toxic shock syndrome
TUR, TURP	transurethral resection of the prostate
TVH	total vaginal hysterectomy
Tx	treatment
U	unit
UA	urinalysis
UAO	upper airway obstruction
UC	uterine contractions

Abbreviations *Continued*

UE	upper extremity
UGI	upper gastrointestinal
umb.	navel *(umbilicus)*
U/O	urinary output
URI	upper respiratory infection
U/S	ultrasound
UTI	urinary tract infection
UV	ultraviolet
VA	visual acuity
VATS	video-assisted thoracoscopy
VC	vital capacity (of lungs)
VCUG	voiding cystourethrogram
VDRL	test for syphilis (venereal disease research laboratory)
VEGF	vascular endothelial growth factor
VF	visual field
vis à vis	as compared with; in relation to
V/Q scan	ventilation-perfusion scan
V/S	vital signs; versus
VSD	ventricular septal defect
VT	ventricular tachycardia (abnormal heart rhythm)
VTE	venous thromboembolism
WAIS	Wechsler Adult Intelligence Scale
WBC, wbc	white blood cell; white blood count
WDWN	well developed, well nourished
WISC	Wechsler Intelligence Scale for Children
WNL	within normal limits
wt	weight
XRT	radiation therapy
y/o, yrs	year(s) old

Symbols*

=	equal
≠	unequal
+	positive
−	negative
↑	above, increase
↓	below, decrease
♀	female
♂	male
→	to (in direction of)
>	is greater than
<	is less than
1°	primary to
2°	secondary to
ʒ	dram
℥	ounce
%	percent
°	degree; hour
:	ratio; "is to"
±	plus or minus (either positive or negative)
′	foot
″	inch
∴	therefore
@	at, each
c̄	with
s̄	without
#	pound
≅	approximately, about
Δ	change
p	short arm of a chromosome
q	long arm of a chromosome

*From Chabner D-E: The Language of Medicine, 7th ed. Philadelphia, WB Saunders, 2004.

Acronyms*

An acronym is the name for an abbreviation that forms a pronounceable word.

ACE (ace)	angiotensin-converting enzyme
AIDS (ades)	acquired immune deficiency syndrome
BUN (bun)	blood, urea, nitrogen
CABG (cabbage)	coronary artery bypass graft
CAT (cat)	computerized axial tomography
CPAP (seepap)	continuous positive airway pressure
ELISA (eliza)	enzyme-linked immunosorbent assay
GERD (gerd)	gastroesophageal reflux disease
HIPAA (hipa)	Health Insurance Portability and Accountability Act of 1996
LASER (lazer)	light amplification by stimulated emission of radiation
LASIK (lasik)	laser *in situ* keratomileusis
LEEP (leep)	loop electrocautery excision procedure
MICU (micku)	medical intensive care unit
MUGA (mugah)	multiple-gated acquisition (scan)
NSAID (insayd)	nonsteroidal anti-inflammatory drug
NICU (nicku)	neonatal intensive care unit
PACS (packs)	picture archival communications system
PALS (palz)	pediatric advanced life support
PEEP (peep)	positive end expiratory pressure
PEG (peg)	percutaneous endoscopic gastrostomy

---

*From Chabner D-E: The Language of Medicine, 7th ed. Philadelphia, WB Saunders, 2004.

PERRLA (perlah)	pupils equal, round, reactive to light and accommodation
PET (pet)	positron emission tomography
PICU (picku)	pediatric intensive care unit
PIP (pip)	proximal interphalangeal joint
PUVA (poovah)	psoralen ultratrviolet A
REM (rem)	rapid eye movement
SAD (sad)	seasonal affective disorder
SARS (sarz)	severe acute respiratory syndrome
SERM (serm)	selective estrogen receptor modulator
SIDS (sidz)	sudden infant death syndrome
SMAC (smak)	sequential multiple analyzer computer (blood testing)
SOAP (soap)	subjective, objective, assessment, plan
SPECT (spekt)	single-photon emission computed tomography
TENS (tenz)	transcutaneous electrical nerve stimulation
TRUS (truss)	transrectal ultrasound
TURP (turp)	transurethral resection of the prostate
VATS (vats)	video-assisted thoracoscopy

Plurals*

The rules commonly used to form plurals of medical terms are as follows:

1. For words ending in **a,** retain the **a** and add **e**: Examples:

Singular	*Plural*
vertebra	vertebrae
bursa	bursae
bulla	bullae

2. For words ending in **is**, drop the **is** and add **es**: Examples:

Singular	*Plural*
anastomosis	anastomoses
metastasis	metastases
epiphysis	epiphyses
prosthesis	prostheses
pubis	pubes

3. For words ending in **ix** and **ex**, drop the **ix** or **ex** and add **ices**: Examples:

Singular	*Plural*
apex	apices
varix	varices

4. For words ending in **on**, drop the **on** and add **a**: Examples:

Singular	*Plural*
ganglion	ganglia
spermatozoon	spermatozoa

*From Chabner D-E: The Language of Medicine, 7th ed. Philadelphia, WB Saunders, 2004.

5. For words ending in **um**, drop the **um** and add **a**:
   Examples:

Singular	*Plural*
bacterium	bacteria
diverticulum	diverticula
ovum	ova

6. For words ending in **us**, drop the **us** and add **i**:
   Examples:

Singular	*Plural*
calculus	calculi
bronchus	bronchi
nucleus	nuclei

Two exceptions to this rule are viruses and sinuses.

7. Examples of other plural changes are:

Singular	*Plural*
foramen	foramina
iris	irides
femur	femora
anomaly	anomalies
biopsy	biopsies
adenoma	adenomata

Medical Terms Easily Confused

Health care professionals who have difficulty with the English language may face particular challenges with terms commonly used in a health care setting. The unique application of words may cause confusion. The words and phrases listed below have been identified as frequently causing problems for health care providers. Entries are presented in pairs so that readers may compare and contrast spellings and definitions of words and phrases that are spelled and/or pronounced similarly.

Term	Definition
abduction	moving away from (often dictated as "A-B-DUC-tion")
adduction	moving toward (often dictated as "A-D-DUC-tion")
absorption	taking up or in of a substance
adsorption	attracting and holding substances at the surface
acetic	sour (as vinegar or acetic acid)
acidic	pertaining to an acid; acid-forming
ascitic	pertaining to fluid accumulation in the abdomen (ascites)
asthenic	pertaining to a lack or loss of energy
afferent	carrying toward a center
efferent	carrying away from a center

Term	Definition
alkalosis	increased alkalinity of blood and tissues
ankylosis	condition of joint stiffening or immobilization
ante-	before; in front of
anti-	against
anuresis	retention of urine in the bladder ("condition without urine")
enuresis	involuntary discharge of urine; bed-wetting
aphagia	inability to swallow
aphakia	absence of the lens of the eye (as in extraction of a cataract)
aphasia	inability to speak or inability to comprehend spoken or written language
aplasia	lack of development of an organ or tissue
aura	sensation that precedes a seizure
aural	pertaining to the ear
oral	pertaining to the mouth
auxilliary	giving assistance or support
axillary	pertaining to the armpit
bisect	cut in half
resect	cut out (remove)
transect	cut across
dissect	cut apart or separate
bolus	single large mass or quantity of drug or medication that is administered orally or intravenously
bullous	pertaining to bullae (large blisters)

Term	Definition
caliber	diameter of a canal or tube; diameter of a bullet
calipers	instrument used to measure thickness or diameter of a solid
callous	hard (as the nature of a callus)
callus	thickened or hardened area of the epidermis (skin); network of woven bone formed at the ends of a broken bone
canker sore	ulceration of the mucous membrane of the mouth
chancre	primary lesion of syphilis (SHANK-er)
carotid	artery of the neck
parotid	salivary gland near the ear
cecal	pertaining to the cecum (first part of the colon)
fecal	pertaining to feces (solid wastes)
thecal	pertaining to a sheath or enclosing case
cerebellum	posterior portion of the brain (responsible for balance)
cerebrum	largest part of the brain (responsible for thought, memory, sensations, speech, vision, movement)
cholic	pertaining to bile
colic	pertaining to acute abdominal pain
cirrhosal	pertaining to cirrhosis (liver disease)
scirrhous	pertaining to hard mass or tumor
serosal	pertaining to a serosa (thin membranous covering)

Term	Definition
serous	pertaining to serum (clear portion of blood minus cells and clotting proteins)
cirrhosis	liver disease
xerosis	condition of dryness
CNS	central nervous system
C&S	culture and sensitivity
creatine	high-energy phosphate compound present in muscle
creatinine	nitrogenous waste product excreted in urine
cytotoxin	a poison (toxin) or an antibody with a toxic action on cells
Cytoxan	drug used in chemotherapy
diverticulitis	inflammation of diverticula
diverticulosis	abnormal condition of presence of diverticula
diarrhea	abnormally frequent and loose bowel movements
diuresis	excretion of abnormally high quantity of urine
dysphagia	difficulty in swallowing
dysphasia	difficulty in speaking
dysplasia	abnormal formation (development)
esotropia	inward turning of the eye; cross-eyed
exotropia	outward turning of the eye; wall-eyed

Term	Definition
facial	pertaining to the face
fascial	pertaining to fascia (connective tissue)
faucial	pertaining to the passageway from the mouth to the pharynx
fovea	cup-shaped pit or depression (central section of the retina of the eye)
phobia	persistent, irrational, intense fear
glands	cells that function within secretory or excretory organs
glans	a small, rounded structure, as the *glans penis* (tip of the organ)
graft	tissue implanted from one place to another
graph	instrument to record data
hematoma	collection of blood (bruise)
hepatoma	malignant tumor of the liver
ileac	pertaining to the third part of the small intestine (ileum)
iliac	pertaining to the upper portion of the hip bone (ilium)
ileum	third part of the small intestine
ilium	superior portion of the hip bone
ileus	obstruction of the intestine
inter-	between
infra-	below, beneath
intra-	within
in vitro	within a test tube ("in glass")
in vivo	within a living organism

Term	Definition
labial	pertaining to a lip or lip-like structure
labile	unstable; gliding from point to point
lice	parasites (singular is *louse*)
lyse	to cause disintegration of a substance
malleolus	bony prominence on either side of the ankle joint
malleus	small bone in the middle portion of the ear
mammoplasty	surgical repair of the breast
manoplasty	plastic surgery of the hand
meiosis	type of cell division to form gametes or sex cells (egg and sperm)
miosis	contraction of the pupil of the eye
mitosis	type of cell division resulting in the formation of identical daughter cells
mycosis	abnormal condition of fungi (molds or yeast infection) in the body
miotic	drug that causes contraction of the pupil of the eye
myopic	pertaining to being nearsighted (myopia)
menorrhagia	excessive uterine bleeding during menstruation
metrorrhagia	abnormal uterine bleeding not during menstruation
menometrorrhagia	excessive uterine bleeding at both menstruation and other times

Term	Definition
mucous	pertaining to or resembling mucus
mucus	secretion from mucous membranes
myeloma	malignant tumor of the bone marrow
myoma	benign tumor of muscle
palpable	able to be felt with a hand
palpebral	pertaining to the eyelid
palpation	touch, feel, and/or examine with hands and fingers
palpitation	rapid pulsation of the heart
perineal	pertaining to the perineum (genital area in female and male)
peritoneal	pertaining to the peritoneum (membrane surrounding abdominal organs)
peroneal	pertaining to the fibula (smaller of two lower leg bones)
pheresis	removal of blood from a donor with a portion separated and retained and the remainder reinfused into the donor; apheresis
-phoresis	indicating transmission (as in electrophoresis or transmission of electricity to separate substances)
pleural	pertaining to pleura (membranes surrounding lungs)
plural	more than one

Term	Definition
pleuritis	inflammation of the pleura
pruritus	itching
prostate	gland at the base of the urinary bladder in males
prostrate	in a horizontal position; lying down
prostatic	pertaining to the prostate gland
prosthetic	pertaining to an artificial device or prosthesis (replacement of a body part)
ureter	one of two tubes each leading from a kidney to the urinary bladder
urethra	tube leading from the urinary bladder to the outside of the body
vesical	pertaining to the urinary bladder
vesicle	a small blister

Definitions of Diagnostic Tests and Procedures*

Radiology, Ultrasound, and Imaging Procedures

In many of the following procedures a *contrast* substance (sometimes referred to as a *dye*) is introduced into or around a body part so that the part can be viewed while x-rays are taken. The contrast substance (often containing barium or iodine) appears dense on the x-ray and outlines the body part that it fills.

The suffix -GRAPHY, meaning "process of recording," is used in many terms describing imaging procedures. The suffix -GRAM, meaning "record," is also used and describes the actual image that is produced by this procedure.

Pronunciation of each term is given with its meaning. The syllable that gets the accent is in **CAPITAL LETTERS.** *Italicized* terms indicate important additional terminology, and terms in SMALL CAPITAL LETTERS are defined elsewhere in this section.

ANGIOGRAPHY (an-je-OG-rah-fe) or **ANGIOGRAM (AN-JE-O-GRAM):** X-ray recording of blood vessels. A contrast substance is injected into blood vessels (veins and arteries), and x-ray pictures are taken of the vessels. In *cerebral angiography*, x-ray pictures are taken of blood vessels in the brain. Angiography is used to detect abnormalities in blood vessels, such as blockage, malformation, and arteriosclerosis. Angiography is performed

---

*From Chabner D-E: Medical Terminology: A Short Course, 3rd ed. Philadelphia, WB Saunders, 2003.

most frequently to view arteries and is often used interchangeably with *arteriography.*

ARTERIOGRAPHY (ar-ter-e-OG-rah-fe) or **ARTERI-OGRAM (ar-TER-e-oh-gram):** X-ray recording of arteries after injection of a contrast substance into an artery. *Coronary arteriography* is the visualization of arteries that bring blood to the heart muscle.

BARIUM TESTS (BAH-re-um tests): X-ray examinations using a liquid barium mixture to locate disorders in the esophagus *(esophagogram),* duodenum, small intestine *(small bowel follow-through),* and colon *(barium enema).* Taken before or during the examination, barium causes the intestinal tract to stand out in silhouette when viewed through a *fluoroscope* or seen on an x-ray film. The *barium swallow* is used to examine the upper gastrointestinal tract, and the *barium enema* is for examination of the lower gastrointestinal tract.

BARIUM ENEMA: See LOWER GASTROINTESTINAL EXAMINATION and BARIUM TESTS.

BARIUM SWALLOW: See ESOPHAGOGRAPHY and BARIUM TESTS.

CARDIAC CATHETERIZATION (KAR-de-ak cath-eh-ter-i-ZA-shun): Procedure in which a catheter (tube) is passed via vein or artery into the chambers of the heart to measure the blood flow out of the heart and the pressures and oxygen content in the heart chambers. Contrast material is also introduced into heart chambers, and x-ray images are taken to show heart structure.

CAT SCAN, CT SCAN: See COMPUTED TOMOGRAPHY.

CEREBRAL ANGIOGRAPHY: See ANGIOGRAPHY.

CHEST X-RAY: An x-ray of the chest that may show infection (as in pneumonia or tuberculosis), emphysema, occupational exposure (asbestosis), lung tumors, or heart enlargement.

CHOLANGIOGRAPHY (kol-an-je-OG-rah-fe) or **CHOLANGIOGRAM (kol-AN-je-o-gram):** X-ray recording of bile ducts. Contrast material is given by intravenous injection *(I.V. cholangiogram)* and collects in the gallbladder and bile ducts. Also, contrast can be introduced (through the skin) by a percutaneously placed needle inserted into an intrahepatic duct *(percutaneous transhepatic cholangiography)*. X-rays are taken of bile ducts to identify obstructions caused by tumors or stones.

COMPUTED TOMOGRAPHY (CT SCAN or **CAT SCAN) (kom-PU-ted to-MOG-ra-fe):** X-ray images taken to show the body in cross-section. Contrast material may be used (injected into the bloodstream) to highlight structures such as the liver, brain, or blood vessels, and barium can be swallowed to outline gastrointestinal organs. X-ray images, taken as the x-ray tube rotates around the body, are processed by a computer to show "slices" of body tissues, most often within the head, chest, and abdomen.

CORONARY ARTERIOGRAPHY: See ARTERIOGRAPHY.

CYSTOGRAPHY (sis-TOG-rah-fe) or **CYSTOGRAM (SIS-to-gram):** X-ray recording of the urinary bladder using a contrast medium so that the outline of the urinary bladder can be seen clearly. A contrast substance is injected via catheter into the urethra and urinary bladder, and x-ray images are taken. A *voiding cystourethrogram* is an x-ray image of the urinary tract made while the patient is urinating.

DIGITAL SUBTRACTION ANGIOGRAPHY (DIJ-i-tal sub-TRAK-shun an-je-OG-rah-fe): A unique x-ray technique for viewing blood vessels by taking two images and subtracting one from the other. Images are first taken without contrast and then again after contrast is injected into blood vessels. The first image is then subtracted from the second so that the final image (sharp and precise) shows only contrast-filled blood vessels minus surrounding tissue.

DOPPLER ULTRASOUND (DOP-ler UL-tra-sound): An instrument focuses sound waves on blood vessels and measures blood flow as echoes bounce off red blood cells. Arteries or veins in the arms, neck, or legs are examined to detect vascular occlusion (blockage) caused by clots or atherosclerosis.

ECHOCARDIOGRAPHY (eh-ko-kar-de-OG-rah-fe) or **ECHOCARDIOGRAM (eh-ko-KAR-de-o-gram):** Images of the heart produced by introducing high-frequency sound waves through the chest into the heart. The sound waves are reflected back from the heart, and echoes showing heart structure are displayed on a recording machine. It is a highly useful diagnostic tool in the evaluation of diseases of the valves that separate the heart chambers and diseases of the heart muscle.

ECHOENCEPHALOGRAPHY (eh-ko-en-sef-ah-LOG-rah-fe) or **ECHOENCEPHALOGRAM (eh-ko-en-SEF-ah-lo-gram):** An ultrasound recording of the brain. Sound waves are beamed at the brain, and the echoes that return to the machine are recorded as graphic tracings. Brain tumors and hematomas can be detected by abnormal tracings.

ENDOSCOPIC RETROGRADE CHOLANGIOPAN-CREATOGRAPHY or **ERCP (en-do-SKOP-ik REH-tro-grad kol-an-je-o-pan-kre-ah-TOG-rah-fe):** X-ray recording of the bile ducts, pancreas, and pancreatic duct. Radiopaque contrast is injected via a tube through the mouth into the bile and pancreatic ducts, and x-rays are then taken.

ESOPHAGOGRAPHY (eh-sof-ah-GOG-rah-fe) or **ESOPHAGOGRAM (eh-SOF-ah-go-gram):** X-ray images taken of the esophagus after barium sulfate is swallowed. This test is also called a *barium meal* or *barium swallow* and is part of an UPPER GAS-TROINTESTINAL EXAMINATION.

FLUOROSCOPY (flur-OS-ko-pe): An x-ray procedure that uses a fluorescent screen rather than a photographic plate to show images of the body. X-rays that have passed through the body strike a screen covered with a fluorescent substance that emits yellow-green light. Internal organs are seen directly and in motion. Fluoroscopy is used to guide the insertion of catheters and during BARIUM TESTS.

GALLBLADDER ULTRASOUND (GAWL-blah-der UL-tra-sownd): Procedure in which sound waves are used to visualize gallstones. This procedure has

replaced cholecystography, which required inges-
tion of an iodine-based contrast substance.

HYSTEROSALPINGOGRAPHY (his-ter-o-sal-ping-OG-rah-fe) or **HYSTEROSALPINGOGRAM (his-ter-o-sal-PING-o-gram):** X-ray recording of the uterus and
fallopian tubes. Contrast medium is inserted through
the vagina into the uterus and fallopian tubes, and x-
rays are taken to detect blockage or tumor.

INTRAVENOUS PYELOGRAPHY: See UROGRAPHY.

**LOWER GASTROINTESTINAL EXAMINATION
(LO-wer gas-tro-in-TES-tin-al ek-zam-ih-NA-
shun):** X-ray pictures of the colon taken after a
liquid contrast substance called barium sulfate is
inserted through a plastic tube (enema) into the
rectum and large intestine (colon). If tumor is
present in the colon, it may appear as an obstruction or irregularity. Also known as a *barium
enema*.

**MAGNETIC RESONANCE IMAGING (mag-NET-ik
REZ-o-nans IM-a-jing)** or **MRI:** Magnetic waves
and radiofrequency pulses, not x-rays, used to
create an image of body organs. The images can
be taken in several planes of the body—frontal,
sagittal (side), and transverse (cross-section)—
and are particularly useful for studying tumors of
the brain and spinal cord. Magnetic waves
beamed at the heart give information about con-
genital heart disease and cardiac lesions before
surgery.

MAMMOGRAPHY (MAMOG-rah-fe) or **MAMMO-
GRAM (MAM-o-gram):** X-ray recording of the
breast. X-rays of low voltage are beamed at the
breast, and images are produced. Mammography is
used to detect abnormalities in breast tissue, such
as early breast cancer.

MYELOGRAPHY (mi-eh-LOG-rah-fe) or **MYELO-
GRAM (MI-eh-lo-gram):** X-ray recording of the
spinal cord. X-rays are taken of the fluid-filled
space surrounding the spinal cord after a contrast
medium is injected into the subarachnoid space
(between the membranes surrounding the spinal

cord) at the lumbar level of the back. Myelography detects tumors or ruptured, "slipped," disks that lie between the backbones (vertebrae) and press on the spinal cord.

PYELOGRAPHY or **PYELOGRAM:** See UROGRAPHY.

SMALL BOWEL FOLLOW-THROUGH: See BARIUM TESTS and UPPER GASTROINTESTINAL EXAMINATION.

TOMOGRAPHY (to-MOG-rah-fe) or **TOMOGRAM (TO-mo-gram):** X-ray recording that shows an organ in depth. Several pictures ("slices") are taken of an organ by moving the x-ray tube and film in sequence to blur out certain regions and bring others into sharper focus. Tomograms of the kidney and lung are examples.

ULTRASONOGRAPHY (ul-trah-so-NOG-rah-fe) or **ULTRASONOGRAM (ul-trah-SON-o-gram):** Images produced by beaming sound waves into the body and capturing the echoes that bounce off organs. These echoes are then processed to produce an image showing the difference between fluid and solid masses and the general position of organs.

UPPER GASTROINTESTINAL EXAMINATION (UP-er gas-tro-in-TES-tin-al ek-zam-ih-NA-shun): X-ray pictures taken of the esophagus *(barium meal* or *barium swallow)*, duodenum, and small intestine after a liquid contrast substance called barium sulfate is swallowed. In a *small bowel follow-through,* pictures are taken at increasing time intervals to follow the progress of barium through the small intestine. Identification of obstructions or ulcers is possible.

UROGRAPHY (u-ROG-rah-fe) or **UROGRAM (UR-o-gram):** X-ray recording of the kidney and urinary tract. If x-rays are taken after contrast medium is injected intravenously, the procedure is called *intravenous urography (descending* or *excretion urography)* or *intravenous pyelography (IVP).* If x-rays are taken after injection of contrast medium into the bladder through the urethra, the procedure is *retrograde urography* or *retrograde pyelography.* PYEL/O- means "renal pelvis" (the collecting chamber of the kidney).

Nuclear Medicine Scans

In the following diagnostic tests, radioactive material *(radioisotope)* is injected, inhaled, or swallowed and then detected by a scanning device in the organ in which it accumulates. X-rays, ultrasound, or magnetic waves are not used.

The pronunciation of each term is given with its meaning. The syllable that gets the accent is in **CAPITAL LETTERS.**

BONE SCAN: Procedure in which a radioactive substance is injected intravenously and its uptake in bones is detected by a scanning device. Tumors in bone can be detected by increased uptake of the radioactive material in the areas of the lesions.

BRAIN SCAN: Procedure in which a radioactive substance is injected intravenously. It collects in any lesion that disturbs the natural barrier that exists between blood vessels and normal brain tissue (blood-brain barrier), allowing the radioactive substance to enter the brain tissue. A scanning device detects the presence of the radioactive substance and thus can identify an area of tumor, abscess, or hematoma.

GALLIUM SCAN (GAL-le-um skan): Procedure in which radioactive gallium (gallium citrate) is injected into the bloodstream and is detected in the body using a scanning device that produces an image of the areas where gallium collects. The gallium collects in areas of certain tumors (Hodgkin disease, hematoma, various adenocarcinomas) and in areas of infection.

MUGA SCAN (MUH-gah skan): Test that uses radioactive technetium to detect a heart attack (myocardial infarction). Also called multiple-gated acquisition scan.

POSITRON EMISSION TOMOGRAPHY (POS-i-tron e-MISH-un to-MOG-rah-fe) or **PET SCAN:** Procedure in which radioactive substances (oxygen and glucose are used) that release radioactive particles called positrons are injected into the body and travel to specialized areas such as the brain and heart. Because of the way that the positrons are released, cross-sectional color pictures can be made showing the location of the radioactive substance. This test is used to study disorders of the brain and to diagnose strokes, epilepsy, schizophrenia, coronary artery disease, and migraine headaches.

PULMONARY PERFUSION SCAN (PUL-mo-ner-e per-FU-shun skan): Procedure in which radioactive particles are injected intravenously and travel rapidly to areas of the lung that are adequately filled with blood. Regions of obstructed blood flow caused by tumor, blood clot, swelling, and inflammation can be seen as nonradioactive areas on the scan.

PULMONARY VENTILATION SCAN (PUL-mo-ner-e ven-ti-LA-shun skan): Procedure in which radioactive gas is inhaled and a special camera detects its presence in the lungs. The scan is used to detect lung segments that fail to fill with the radioactive gas. Lack of filling is usually due to diseases that obstruct the bronchial tubes and air sacs. This scan is also used in the evaluation of lung function before surgery.

TECHNETIUM 99m SESTABIBI SCAN (tek-NE-she-um 99m ses-tah-MIH-be skan): A radioisotope (technetium and sestabibi) is injected intravenously and used to define areas of poor blood flow in heart muscle. This scan is also used with an *exercise tolerance test (ETT-MIBI)*.

THALLIUM-201 SCAN (THAL-e-um-201 skan): Procedure in which thallium-201 is injected into a vein and images of blood flow through heart muscle are recorded as a person performs an exercise test.

THYROID SCAN (THI-royd skan): Procedure in which a radioactive iodine chemical is injected intravenously and collects in the thyroid gland. A scanning device detects the radioactive substance in the gland, measuring it and producing an image of the gland. The increased or decreased activity of the gland is demonstrated by the gland's capacity to use the radioactive iodine. A thyroid scan is used to evaluate the position, size, and functioning of the thyroid gland.

Clinical Procedures

The following procedures are performed on patients to establish a correct diagnosis of an abnormal condition. In some instances, the procedure may also be used to treat the condition.

Pronunciation of each term is given with its meaning. The syllable that gets the accent is in **CAPITAL LETTERS.** Terms in SMALL CAPITAL LETTERS are defined elsewhere in this section. *Italicized* terms are additional important terminology.

ABDOMINOCENTESIS (ab-dom-in-o-sen-TE-sis): See PARACENTESIS.

AMNIOCENTESIS (am-ne-o-sen-TE-sis): Surgical puncture to remove fluid from the sac (amnion) that surrounds the fetus in the uterus. The fluid contains cells from the fetus that can be examined under a microscope for chromosomal analysis.

ASPIRATION (as-peh-RA-shun): The withdrawal of fluid by suction through a needle or tube. The term "aspiration pneumonia" refers to an infection caused by inhalation into the lungs of food or an object.

AUDIOMETRY (aw-de-OM-eh-tre): A test using sound waves of various frequencies (e.g., 500 Hz) up to 8000 Hz, which quantifies the extent and type of hearing loss. An *audiogram* is the record produced by this test.

AUSCULTATION (aw-skul-TA-shun): The process of listening for sounds produced within the body. This is most often performed with the aid of a stethoscope to determine the condition of the chest or abdominal organs or to detect the fetal heart beat.

BIOPSY (BI-op-se): The removal of a piece of tissue from the body and subsequent examination of the tissue under a microscope. The procedure is performed by means of a surgical knife, by needle aspiration, or via endoscopic removal (using a special forceps-like instrument inserted through a hollow flexible tube). An *excisional biopsy* means that the entire tissue to be examined is removed. An *incisional biopsy* is the removal of only a small amount of tissue, and a *needle biopsy* indicates that tissue is pierced with a hollow needle and fluid is withdrawn for microscopic examination.

BONE MARROW BIOPSY (bon MAH-ro BI-op-se): The removal of a small amount of bone marrow. The cells are then examined under a microscope. Often the hip bone (iliac crest) is used, and the biopsy is helpful in determining the number and type of blood cells in the bone marrow. Also called a bone marrow ASPIRATION.

BRONCHOSCOPY (brong-KOS-ko-pe): The insertion of a flexible tube (endoscope) into the airway. The lining of the bronchial tubes can be seen, and tissue may be removed for biopsy. The tube is usually inserted through the mouth but can also be directly inserted into the airway during MEDIASTINOSCOPY. Sedation is required for this procedure.

CHORIONIC VILLUS SAMPLING (kor-e-ON-ik VIL-us SAM-pling): Removal and microscopic analysis of a small piece of placental tissue to detect fetal abnormalities.

COLONOSCOPY (ko-lon-OS-ko-pe): The insertion of a flexible tube (endoscope) through the rectum into the colon for visual examination. Biopsy samples may be taken and benign growths, such as polyps, can be removed through the endoscope. The removal of a polyp is called a *polypectomy* (pol-eh-PEK-to-me).

COLPOSCOPY (kol-POS-ko-pe): The inspection of the cervix through the insertion of a special microscope into the vagina. The vaginal walls are held apart by a speculum so that the cervix (entrance to the uterus) can come into view.

CONIZATION (ko-nih-ZA-shun): The removal of a cone-shaped sample of uterine cervix tissue. This sample is then examined under a microscope for evidence of cancerous growth. The special shape of the tissue sample allows the pathologist to examine the transitional zone of the cervix, where cancers are most likely to develop.

CULDOCENTESIS (kul-do-sen-TE-sis): The insertion of a thin, hollow needle through the vagina into the cul-de-sac, the space between the rectum and the uterus. Fluid is withdrawn and analyzed for evidence of cancerous cells, infection, or blood cells.

CYSTOSCOPY (sis-TOS-ko-pe): The insertion of a thin tube or cystoscope (endoscope) into the urethra and then into the urinary bladder to visualize the bladder. A biopsy of the urinary bladder can be performed through the cystoscope.

DIGITAL RECTAL EXAMINATION (DIG-ih-tal REK-tal eks-am-ih-NA-shun): Procedure in which the physician inserts a gloved finger into the rectum. This procedure is used to detect rectal cancer and as a primary method of detection of prostate cancer. The abbreviation is *DRG*.

DILATION AND CURETTAGE (di-LA-shun and kur-ih-TAJ): Procedure in which a series of probes of increasing size is systematically inserted through the vagina into the opening of the cervix. The cervix is thus dilated (widened) so that a curette (spoon-shaped instrument) can be inserted to remove tissue from the lining of the uterus. The tissue is then examined under a microscope. The abbreviation for this procedure is *D&C*.

ELECTROCARDIOGRAPHY (e-lek-tro-kar-de-OG-rah-fe): The connection of electrodes (wires or "leads") to the body to record electric impulses from the heart. The *electrocardiogram* is the actual record produced, and it is useful in discovering abnormalities in heart rhythms and diagnosing heart disorders. The abbreviation is *EKG* or *ECG*.

ELECTROENCEPHALOGRAPHY (e-lek-tro-en-sef-ah-LOG-rah-fe): The connection of electrodes (wires or "leads") to the scalp to record electricity coming from within the brain. The *electroencephalogram* is the actual record produced. It is useful in the diagnosis and monitoring of epilepsy and other brain lesions and in the investigation of neurological disorders. It is also used to evaluate patients in coma (brain inactivity) and in the study of sleep disorders. The abbreviation is *EEG*.

ELECTROMYOGRAPHY (e-lek-tro-mi-OG-rah-fe):
The insertion of needle electrodes into muscle to record electrical activity. This procedure detects injuries and diseases that affect muscles and nerves. The abbreviation is *EMG*.

ENDOSCOPY (en-DOS-ko-pe): The insertion of a thin, tube-like instrument (endoscope) into an organ or cavity. The endoscope is placed through a natural opening (the mouth or anus) or into a surgical incision, such as through the abdominal wall. Endoscopes contain bundles of glass fibers that carry light (fiberoptic); some instruments are equipped with a small forceps-like device that withdraws a sample of tissue for microscopic study (biopsy). Examples of endoscopy are BRONCHOSCOPY, COLONOSCOPY, ESOPHAGOSCOPY, GASTROSCOPY, and LAPAROSCOPY.

ESOPHAGOGASTRODUODEN3OSCOPY (eh-SOF-ah-go-GAS-tro-du-o-den-NOS-ko-pe): The insertion of an endoscope through the mouth into the esophagus, stomach, and first part of the small intestine. Also called *EGD*.

ESOPHAGOSCOPY (eh-sof-ah-GOS-ko-pe): The insertion of an endoscope through the mouth and throat into the esophagus. Visual examination of the esophagus to detect ulcers, tumors, or other lesions is thus possible.

EXCISIONAL BIOPSY (ek-SIZZ-in-al BI-op-se): See BIOPSY.

FROZEN SECTION (FRO-zen SEK-shun): The quick preparation of a biopsy sample for examination during an actual surgical procedure. Tissue is taken from the operating room to the pathology laboratory and frozen. It is then thinly sliced and immediately examined under a microscope to determine if the sample is benign or malignant and to determine the status of margins.

GASTROSCOPY (gas-TROS-ko-pe): The insertion of an endoscope through the esophagus into the stomach for visual examination and/or biopsy of the stomach. When the upper portion of the small intestine is also visualized, the procedure is called *EGD* or ESOPHAGOGASTRODUODENOSCOPY.

HOLTER MONITOR (HOL-ter ECG MON-ih-ter): The electrocardiographic record of heart activity over an extended period of time. The Holter monitor is worn by the patient as he/she performs normal daily activities. It detects and aids in the management of heart rhythm abnormalities. Also called *ambulatory electrocardiograph.*

HYSTEROSCOPY (his-ter-OS-ko-pe): The insertion of an endoscope into the uterus for visual examination.

INCISIONAL BIOPSY (in-SIZZ-in-al BI-op-se): See BIOPSY.

LAPAROSCOPY (lap-ah-ROS-ko-pe): The insertion of an endoscope into the abdomen. After the patient receives a local anesthetic, a laparoscope is inserted through an incision in the abdominal wall. This procedure gives the doctor a view of the abdominal cavity, the surface of the liver and spleen, and the pelvic region. Laparoscopy is used to perform fallopian tube ligation as a means of preventing pregnancy.

LARYNGOSCOPY (lah-rin-GOS-ko-pe): The insertion of an endoscope into the airway to visually examine the voice box (larynx). A laryngoscope transmits a magnified image of the larynx through a system of lenses and mirrors. The procedure can reveal tumors and explain changes in the voice. Sputum samples and tissue biopsies are obtained by using brushes or forceps attached to the laryngoscope.

MEDIASTINOSCOPY (me-de-ah-sti-NOS-ko-pe): The insertion of an endoscope into the mediastinum (space in the chest between the lungs and in front of the heart). A mediastinoscope is inserted through a small incision in the neck while the patient is under anesthesia. This procedure is used to biopsy lymph nodes and to examine other structures within the mediastinum.

NEEDLE BIOPSY (NE-dl BI-op-se): See BIOPSY.

OPHTHALMOSCOPIC EXAM (of-thal-mo-SKOP-ic ek-ZAM): A physician uses an *ophthalmoscope* to look directly into the eye, evaluating the optic nerve, retina, and blood vessels in the back of the eye and the lens in the front of the eye for cataracts. Also called *ophthalmoscopy.*

OTOSCOPIC EXAM (o-to-SKOP-ic ek-ZAM): A physician uses an *otoscope* inserted into the ear canal to check for obstructions (e.g., wax), infection, fluid, and eardrum perforations or scarring. Also called *otoscopy.*

PALPATION (pal-PA-shun): Examination by touch. This is a technique of manual physical examination by which a doctor feels underlying tissues and organs through the skin.

PAP SMEAR (pap smer): The insertion of a cotton swab or wooden spatula into the vagina to obtain a sample of cells from the outer surface of the cervix (neck of the uterus). The cells are then smeared on a glass slide, preserved, and sent to the laboratory for microscopic examination. This test for cervical cancer was developed and named after the late Dr. George Papanicolaou. Results are reported as a Grade I to IV (I = normal, II = inflammatory, III = suspicious of malignancy, IV = malignancy).

PARACENTESIS (pah-rah-sen-TE-sis): Surgical puncture of the membrane surrounding the abdomen (peritoneum) to remove fluid from the abdominal cavity. Fluid is drained for analysis and to prevent its accumulation in the abdomen. Also known as *abdominocentesis.*

PELVIC EXAM (PEL-vik ek-ZAM): Physician examines female sex organs and checks the uterus and ovaries for enlargement, cysts, tumors, or abnormal bleeding. This is also known as an "internal exam."

PERCUSSION (per-KUSH-un): The technique of striking a part of the body with short, sharp taps of the fingers to determine the size, density, and position of the underlying parts by the sound obtained. Percussion is commonly used on the abdomen to examine the liver.

PROCTOSIGMOIDOSCOPY (prok-to-sig-moy-DOS-ko-pe): The insertion of an endoscope through the anus to examine the first 10 to 12 inches of the rectum and colon. When the sigmoid colon is visualized using a longer endoscope, the procedure is called *sigmoidoscopy.* The procedure detects polyps, malignant tumors, and sources of bleeding.

PULMONARY FUNCTION TEST (PUL-mo-ner-e FUNG-shun test): The measurement of the air taken into and exhaled from the lungs by means of an instrument called a *spirometer.* The test may be abnormal in patients with asthma, chronic bronchitis, emphysema, and occupational exposures to asbestos, chemicals, and dusts.

SIGMOIDOSCOPY (sig-moy-DOS-ko-pe): See PROCTOSIGMOIDOSCOPY.

STRESS TEST (stres TEST): An electrocardiogram taken during exercise. It may reveal hidden heart disease or confirm the cause of cardiac symptoms.

THORACENTESIS (thor-ah-sen-TE-sis): The insertion of a needle into the chest to remove fluid from the space surrounding the lungs (pleural cavity). After injection of a local anesthetic, a hollow needle is placed through the skin and muscles of the back and into the space between the lungs and chest wall. Fluid is then withdrawn by applying suction. Excess fluid *(pleural effusion)* may be a sign of infection or malignancy. This procedure is used to diagnose conditions, to drain a pleural effusion, or to re-expand a collapsed lung *(atelectasis).*

THORASCOPY (tho-RAS-ko-pe): The insertion of an endoscope through an incision in the chest to visually examine the surface of the lungs. Also called *thoracoscopy.*

Laboratory Tests

The following laboratory tests are performed on samples of a patient's blood, *plasma* (fluid portion of the blood), *serum* (plasma minus clotting proteins and produced after blood has clotted), urine, feces, *sputum* (mucus coughed up from the lungs), *cerebrospinal fluid* (fluid within the spaces around the spinal cord and brain), and skin.

Pronunciation of each term is given with its meaning. The syllable that gets the accent is in **CAPITAL LETTERS.** Terms in SMALL CAPITAL LETTERS are defined elsewhere in this section. *Italicized* terms are additional important terminology.

ACID PHOSPHATASE (AH-sid FOS-fah-tas): Measurement of the amount of an enzyme called *acid phosphatase* in serum. Enzyme levels are elevated in metastatic prostate cancer. Moderate elevations of this enzyme occur in diseases of bone and when breast cancer cells invade bone tissue.

ALBUMIN (al-BU-min): Measurement of the amount of albumin (protein) in both the serum and the urine. A decrease of albumin in serum indicates disease of the kidneys, malnutrition, or liver disease or may occur in extensive loss of protein in the gut or from the skin, as in a burn. The presence of albumin in the urine *(albuminuria)* indicates malfunction of the kidney.

ALKALINE PHOSPHATASE (AL-kah-lin FOS-fah-tas): Measurement of the amount of *alkaline phosphatase* (an enzyme found on cell membranes) in serum. Levels are elevated in liver diseases (such as hepatitis and hepatoma) and in bone disease and bone cancer. The laboratory symbol is *alk phos.*

ALPHA-FETOPROTEIN (al-fa-fe-to-PRO-teen): Determination of the presence of a protein called alpha-globulin in serum. The protein is normally present in the serum of the fetus, infant, and pregnant woman. In fetuses with abnormalities of the brain and spinal cord, the protein leaks into the amniotic fluid surrounding the fetus and is an indicator of spinal tube defect (spina bifida) or anencephaly (lack of brain development). High levels are found in patients with cancer of the liver and other malignancies (testicular and ovarian cancers). Serum levels monitor the effectiveness of cancer treatment. Elevated levels are also seen in benign liver disease such as cirrhosis and viral hepatitis. The laboratory symbol is *AFP.*

ALT: Measurement of the amount of the enzyme called *alanine transaminase* in serum. The enzyme is normally present in blood but accumulates in high amounts with damage to liver cells. Also called *SGPT.*

ANA: See ANTINUCLEAR ANTIBODY TEST.

ANTINUCLEAR ANTIBODY TEST (an-tih-NU-kle-ar AN-tih-bod-e test): Procedure in which a sample of plasma is tested for the presence of antibodies that are found in patients with systemic lupus erythematosus. Laboratory symbol is *ANA.*

AST: Measurement of the enzyme *aspartate transaminase* in serum. The enzyme is normally present in blood but accumulates when there is damage to the heart or to liver cells. Also called *SGOT.*

BENCE JONES PROTEIN (BENS jonz PRO-teen): Measurement of the presence of the Bence Jones protein in serum or urine. Bence Jones protein is a fragment of a normal serum protein, an immunoglobulin, produced by cancerous bone marrow cells (myeloma cells). Normally it is not found in either blood or urine, but in *multiple myeloma* (a malignant condition of bone marrow) high levels of Bence Jones protein are detected in urine and serum.

BILIRUBIN (bil-ih-RU-bin): Measurement of the amount of bilirubin, a yellow to orange bile pigment, in serum and urine. Bilirubin is derived from hemoglobin, the oxygen-carrying protein in red blood cells. Its presence in high concentration in serum and urine causes *jaundice* (yellow coloration of the skin) and may indicate disease of the liver, obstruction of bile ducts, or a type of anemia that leads to excessive destruction of red blood cells.

BLOOD CHEMISTRY PROFILE: A comprehensive blood test that is a biochemical examination of various substances in the blood using a computerized laboratory analyzer. Tests include calcium (bones), phosphorus (bones), urea (kidney), creatinine (kidney), bilirubin (liver), AST or SGOT (liver and heart muscle) and ALT or SGPT (liver), alkaline phosphatase (liver and bone), globulin (liver and immune disorders), and albumin (liver and kidney). Also called SMA or sequential multiple analysis. SMA-6, SMA-12, and SMA-18 indicate the number of blood elements tested.

BLOOD CULTURE (blud KUL-chur): Test to determine whether infection is present in the bloodstream. A sample of blood is added to a special medium (food) that promotes the growth of microorganisms. The medium is then examined by a medical technologist for evidence of bacteria or other microbes.

BLOOD UREA NITROGEN (blud u-RE-ah NI-tro-jen): Measurement of the amount of urea (nitrogen-containing waste material) in serum. A high level of serum urea indicates poor kidney function, since it is the kidney's job to remove urea from the bloodstream and filter it into urine. The laboratory symbol is *BUN*.

CALCIUM (KAL-se-um): Measurement of the amount of calcium in serum, plasma, or whole blood. Low blood levels are associated with abnormal functioning of nerves and muscles, and high blood levels indicate loss of calcium from bones, excessive intake of calcium, disease of the parathyroid glands, or cancer. The laboratory symbol is *Ca*.

CARBON DIOXIDE (KAR-bon di-OK-side): Blood test to measure the gas produced in tissues and eliminated by the lungs. Abnormal levels may reflect lung disorders. The laboratory symbol is CO_2.

CARCINOEMBRYONIC ANTIGEN (kar-sih-no-em-bree-ON-ik AN-ti-jen): A plasma test for a protein normally found in the blood of human fetuses and produced in healthy adults only in a very small amount, if at all. High levels of this antigen may be a sign of one of a variety of cancers, especially colon or pancreatic cancer. This test is used to monitor the response of patients to cancer treatment. The laboratory abbreviation is *CEA*.

CEREBROSPINAL FLUID (seh-re-bro-SPI-nal FLU-id): Measurement of cerebrospinal fluid for protein, sugar, and blood cells. The fluid is also cultured to detect microorganisms. Chemical tests are performed on specimens of the fluid removed by *lumbar puncture*. Abnormal conditions such as meningitis, brain tumor, and encephalitis are detected. The laboratory abbreviation is *CSF*.

CHOLESTEROL (ko-LES-ter-ol): Measurement of the amount of cholesterol (substance found in animal fats and oils, egg yolks, and milk) in serum or plasma. Normal values vary for age and diet; levels above 200 mg/dl indicate a need for further testing and efforts to reduce cholesterol level, since high levels are associated with hardening of arteries and heart disease. Blood is also tested for the presence of a lipoprotein substance that is a combination of cholesterol and protein. High levels of (optimum level is 60 to 100 mg/dL) *HDL* (high-density lipoprotein) cholesterol in the blood are beneficial, since HDL cholesterol promotes the removal and excretion of excess cholesterol from the body, whereas high levels of low-density lipoprotein *(LDL)* are associated with the development of atherosclerosis (optimum level is 100 mg/dl or less).

COMPLETE BLOOD COUNT: Determinations of the numbers of leukocytes (white blood cells), erythrocytes (red blood cells), and platelets (clotting cells). The CBC is useful in diagnosing anemia, infection, and blood cell disorders, such as leukemia.

CREATINE KINASE (KRE-ah-tin KI-nas): Measurement of levels of creatine kinase, a blood enzyme. Creatine kinase is normally found in heart muscle, brain tissue, and skeletal muscle. The presence of one form *(isoenzyme)* of creatine kinase (either CK-MB or CK2) in the blood is strongly indicative of recent myocardial infarction (heart attack), since the enzyme is released from heart muscle when the muscle is damaged or dying.

CREATININE (kre-AT-ih-neen): Measurement of the amount of creatinine, a nitrogen-containing waste material, in serum or plasma. It is the most reliable test for kidney function. Since creatinine is normally produced as a protein breakdown product in muscle and is excreted by the kidney in urine, an elevation in the creatinine level in the blood indicates a disturbance of kidney function. Elevations are also seen in high-protein diets and dehydration.

CREATININE CLEARANCE (kre-AT-ih-neen KLEER-ans): Measurement of the rate at which creatinine is cleared (filtered) by the kidneys from the blood. A low creatinine clearance indicates that the kidneys are not functioning effectively to clear creatinine from the bloodstream and filter it into urine.

CULTURE (KUL-chur): Identification of microorganisms in a special laboratory medium (fluid, solid, or semisolid material). In *sensitivity* tests, culture plates containing a specific microorganism are prepared, and antibiotic-containing disks are applied to the culture surface. After overnight incubation, the area surrounding the disk (where growth was inhibited) is measured to determine whether the antibiotic is effective against the specific organism.

DIFFERENTIAL (di-fer-EN-shul): See WHITE BLOOD CELL COUNT.

ELECTROLYTES (e-LEK-tro-litz): Determination of the concentration of *electrolytes* (chemical substances capable of conducting an electric current) in serum or whole blood. When dissolved in water, electrolytes break apart into charged particles *(ions)*. The positively charged electrolytes are *sodium* (Na^+), *potassium* (K^+), *calcium* (Ca^{++}), and *magnesium* (Mg^{++}). The negatively charged electrolytes are *chloride* (Cl^-) and *bicarbonate* (HCO_3^-). These charged particles should be present at all times for proper functioning of cells. An electrolyte imbalance occurs when serum concentration is either too high or too low. Calcium balance can affect the bones, kidneys, gastrointestinal tract, and neuromuscular activity, and sodium balance affects blood pressure, nerve functioning, and fluid levels surrounding cells. Potassium balance affects heart and muscular activity.

ELECTROPHORESIS: See SERUM PROTEIN ELECTROPHORESIS.

ELISA (eh-LI-zah): A laboratory assay (test) for the presence of antibodies to the AIDS virus. If a patient tests positive, it is likely that his/her blood contains the AIDS virus (HIV or human immunodeficiency virus). The presence of the virus stimulates white blood cells to make antibodies that are detected by the ELISA assay. This is the first test done to detect AIDS infection and is followed by a WESTERN BLOT test to confirm the results. ELISA is an acronym for *e*nzyme-*l*inked *i*mmuno*s*orbent *a*ssay.

ERYTHROCYTE SEDIMENTATION RATE (eh-RITH-ro-sit sed-ih-men-TA-shun rat): Measurement of the rate at which red blood cells (erythrocytes) in well-mixed venous blood settle to the bottom (sediment) of a test tube. If the rate of sedimentation is markedly slow (elevated sed rate), it may indicate inflammatory conditions, such as rheumatoid arthritis, or conditions that produce excessive proteins in the blood. Laboratory symbols are *ESR* and *sed rate*.

ESTRADIOL (es-tra-DI-ol): A test for the concentration of estradiol, which is a form of estrogen (female hormone) in serum, plasma, or urine.

ESTROGEN RECEPTOR ASSAY (ES-tro-jen re-SEP-tor AS-a): Test, performed at the time of a biopsy, to determine whether a sample of tumor contains an estrogen receptor protein. The protein, if present on breast cancer cells, combines with estrogen, allowing estrogen to promote the growth of the tumor. Thus, if an estrogen receptor assay test is positive (the protein is present), then treatment with an anti-estrogen drug would retard tumor growth. If the assay is negative (the protein is not present), then the tumor would not be affected by anti-estrogen drug treatment.

GLOBULIN (GLOB-u-lin): Measurement (in serum) of proteins that bind to and destroy foreign substances (antigens). Globulins are made by cells of the immune system. *Gamma globulin* is one type of globulin that contains antibodies to fight disease.

GLUCOSE (GLU-kos): Measurement of the amount of glucose (sugar) in serum and plasma. High levels of glucose *(hyperglycemia)* indicate diseases such as diabetes mellitus and hyperthyroidism. Glucose is also measured in urine, and its presence indicates diabetes mellitus.

GLUCOSE TOLERANCE TEST (GLU-kos TOL-erans test): Test to determine how the body uses glucose. In the first part of this test, blood and urine samples are taken after the patient has fasted. Then a solution of glucose is given by mouth. A half hour after the glucose is taken, blood and urine samples are obtained again, and are collected every hour for 4 to 5 hours. This test can indicate abnormal conditions such as diabetes mellitus, hypoglycemia, and liver or adrenal gland dysfunction.

HEMATOCRIT (he-MAT-o-krit): Measurement of the percentage of red blood cells in the blood. The normal range is 40% to 50% in males and 37% to 47% in females. A low hematocrit indicates anemia. The laboratory symbol is *Hct*.

HEMOCCULT TEST (he-mo-o-KULT test): Examination of small sample of stool for otherwise inapparent occult (hidden) traces of blood. The sample is placed on the surface of a collection kit and reacts with a chemical (e.g., guaiac). A positive result may indicate bleeding from polyps, ulcers, or malignant tumors. This is an important screening test for colon cancer. Also called a *stool guaiac test*.

HEMOGLOBIN ASSAY (HE-mo-glo-bin AS-a): Measurement of the concentration of hemoglobin in blood. The normal blood hemoglobin ranges are 13.5 to 18.0 gm/dl in adult males and 12.0 to 16.0 gm/dl in adult females. The laboratory symbol is *Hgb*.

HUMAN CHORIONIC GONADOTROPIN (HU-man kor-e-ON-ik go-nad-o-TRO-pin): Measurement of the concentration of human chorionic gonadotropin (a hormone secreted by cells of the fetal placenta) in urine. It is detected in urine within days after fertilization of egg and sperm cells and provides the basis of the most commonly used pregnancy test. The laboratory symbol is *hCG.*

IMMUNOASSAY (im-u-no-AS-a): A method of testing blood and urine for the concentration of various chemicals, such as hormones, drugs, or proteins. The technique makes use of the immunological reaction between antigens and antibodies. An *assay* is a determination of the amount of any particular substance in a mixture.

LIPID TESTS (LIP-id tests): Lipids are fatty substances such as cholesterol and triglycerides. See CHOLESTEROL and TRIGLYCERIDES.

LIPOPROTEIN TESTS (li-po-PRO-teen tests): See CHOLESTEROL.

LIVER FUNCTION TESTS (LIV-er FUNG-shun tests): See ALKALINE PHOSPHATASE, BILIRUBIN, ALT, and AST.

OCCULT BLOOD TEST: See HEMOCCULT TEST.

PKU TEST: Test that determines whether the urine of a newborn baby contains substances called *phenylketones.* If so, the condition is called *phenylketonuria (PKU).* Phenylketonuria occurs in infants born lacking a specific enzyme. If the enzyme is missing, high levels of *phenylalanine* (an amino acid) accumulate in the blood, affecting the infant's brain and causing mental retardation. This situation is prevented by placing the infant on a special diet that prevents accumulation of phenylalanine in the bloodstream.

PLATELET COUNT (PLAT-let kownt): Determination of the number of clotting cells (platelets) in a sample of blood.

POTASSIUM (po-TAHS-e-um): Measurement of the concentration of potassium in serum. Potassium combines with other minerals (such as calcium) and is an important chemical for proper functioning of muscles, especially the heart muscle. The laboratory symbol is K^+. See also ELECTROLYTES.

PROGESTERONE RECEPTOR ASSAY (pro-JES-teh-rone re-SEP-tor AS-a): Test to determines whether a sample of tumor contains a progesterone receptor protein. A positive test identifies when tumor would be responsive to anti-progesterone hormone therapy.

PROSTATE-SPECIFIC ANTIGEN (PROS-tat speh-SIH-fik AN-tih-jen): Blood test that measures the amount of an antigen elevated in all patients with prostatic cancer and in some with an inflamed prostate gland. The laboratory symbol is *PSA*.

PROTEIN ELECTROPHORESIS: See SERUM PROTEIN ELECTROPHORESIS.

PROTHROMBIN TIME (pro-THROM-bin tim): Measurement of the activity of factors in the blood that participate in clotting. Deficiency of any of these factors can lead to a prolonged pro-thrombin time and difficulty in blood clotting. The test is important as a monitor for patients taking anticoagulants, substances that block the activity of blood clotting factors and increase the risk of bleeding.

PSA: See PROSTATE-SPECIFIC ANTIGEN.

RED BLOOD CELL COUNT: Test to determine the number of erythrocytes in a sample of blood. A low red blood cell count may indicate *anemia*. A high count can indicate *polycythemia vera*.

RHEUMATOID FACTOR (ROO-mah-toyd FAK-tor): Detection of the abnormal protein *rheumatoid factor* in the serum. It is found in patients with rheumatoid arthritis.

SERUM PROTEIN ELECTROPHORESIS (SE-rum PRO-teen e-lek-tro-for-E-sis): A procedure that separates proteins using an electric current. The material tested, such as serum, containing various proteins, is placed on paper or gel or in liquid, and under the influence of an electric current, the proteins separate (-PHORESIS means "separation") so that they can be identified and measured. The procedure is also known as *protein electrophoresis*.

SGOT: See AST.

SGPT: See ALT.

SKIN TESTS: Tests in which substances are applied to the skin or injected under the skin and the reaction of immune cells in the skin is observed. These tests detect a person's sensitivity to substances such as dust or pollen. They can also indicate if a person has been exposed to the bacteria that cause tuberculosis or diphtheria.

SODIUM: See ELECTROLYTES.

SMAC: See BLOOD CHEMISTRY PROFILE.

SPUTUM TEST (SPU-tum test): Examination of mucus coughed up from a patient's lungs. The sputum is examined microscopically and chemically and is cultured for the presence of microorganisms.

STOOL GUAIAC TEST (stool GWI-ak test): See HEMOCCULT TEST.

THYROID FUNCTION TESTS (THI-royd FUNG-shun tests): Tests that measure the levels of thyroid hormones, such as *thyroxine* (T_4) and *triiodothyronine* (T_3), in serum. *Thyroid-stimulating hormone (TSH)*, which is produced by the pituitary gland and stimulates the release of T_4 and T_3 from the thyroid gland, can also be measured in serum. These tests aid in the diagnosis of hypothyroidism and hyperthyroidism and are helpful in monitoring response to thyroid treatment.

TRIGLYCERIDES (tri-GLIS-er-ides): Determination of the amount of *triglycerides* (fats) in the serum. Elevated triglyceride levels are considered an important risk factor for the development of heart disease.

TROPONIN (tro-PO-nin): Measurement of troponin-I and troponin-T in the serum as evidence of a heart attack. Troponin is a protein released into circulation after myocardial (heart muscle) injury.

URIC ACID (UR-ik AS-id): Measurement of the amount of uric acid (a nitrogen-containing waste material) in the serum and urine. High serum levels indicate a type of arthritis called *gout*. In gout, uric acid accumulates as crystals in joints and in tissues. High levels of uric acid may also cause kidney stones.

URINALYSIS (u-rih-NAL-ih-sis): Examination of urine as an aid in the diagnosis of disease. Routine urinalysis involves the observation of unusual color or odor; determination of specific gravity (amount of materials dissolved in urine); chemical tests (for protein, sugar, acetone); and microscopic examination for bacteria, blood cells, and sediment. Urinalysis is used to detect abnormal functioning of the kidneys and bladder, infections, abnormal growths, and diabetes mellitus. The laboratory symbol is *UA*.

WESTERN BLOT (WES-tern blot): Test used to detect infection by *HIV* (AIDS virus). It is more specific than the ELISA. A patient's serum is mixed with purified proteins from HIV, and the reaction is examined. If the patient has made antibodies to HIV, those antibodies will react with the purified HIV proteins, and the test will be positive.

WHITE BLOOD CELL (WBC) COUNT: Determination of the number of leukocytes in the blood. Higher than normal counts can indicate the presence of infection or leukemia. A *differential* is the percentages of different types of white blood cells (neutrophils, eosinophils, basophils, lymphocytes, and monocytes) in a sample of blood. It gives more specific information about leukocytes and aids in the diagnosis of allergic diseases, disorders of the immune system, and various forms of leukemia.

part 2

USEFUL
INFORMATION

Abbreviations for Selected Health Care Organizations, Associations, and Agencies*

AAAA	American Academy of Anesthesiologist's Assistants
AAAAI	American Academy of Allergy, Asthma, and Immunology
AAATP	Association for Anesthesiologist's Assistants Training Program
AAB	American Association of Bioanalysts
AABB	American Association of Blood Banks
AACA	American Association of Clinical Anatomists
AACAHPO	American Association of Certified Allied Health Personnel in Ophthalmology
AACC	American Association for Clinical Chemistry
AACCN	American Association of Critical Care Nurses
AACN	American Association of Colleges of Nursing
AADS	American Association of Dental Schools
AAFP	American Academy of Family Physicians
AAHA	American Academy of Health Administration
AAHC	Association of Academic Health Centers

Chart continued on following page

---

*Modified from Miller-Keane: Encyclopedia & Dictionary Of Medicine, Nursing & Allied Health, 7th ed. Philadelphia, WB Saunders, 2003.

Abbreviatons for Selected Health Care Organizations, Associations, and Agencies
Continued

AAHE	Association for the Advancement of Health Education
AAHP	American Association of Health Planners
AAHPER	American Association for Health, Physical Education, and Recreation
AAMA	American Association of Medical Assistants
AAMC	Association of American Medical Colleges
AAMI	Association for the Advancement of Medical Instrumentation
AAMT	American Association for Music Therapy
AAN	American Academy of Neurology
AAN	American Academy of Nursing
AANA	American Association of Nurse Anesthetists
AAO	American Association of Ophthalmology
AAO	American Association of Orthodontists
AAOHN	American Association of Occupational Health Nurses
AAP	American Academy of Pediatrics
AAPA	American Academy of Physicians Assistants
AAPMR	American Academy of Physical Medicine and Rehabilitation
AARC	American Association for Respiratory Care
AART	American Association for Rehabilitation Therapy
AATA	American Art Therapy Association
AATS	American Association for Thoracic Surgery
ABCP	American Board of Cardiovascular Perfusion

Abbreviations for Selected Health Care Organizations, Associations, and Agencies
Continued

ABNF	Association of Black Nursing Faculty in Higher Education
ACAAI	American College of Asthma, Allergy and Immunology
ACC	American College of Cardiology
ACCP	American College of Chest Physicians
ACEN	Academy of Chief Executive Nurses (Canada)
ACEP	American College of Emergency Physicians
ACHA	American College of Hospital Administrators
ACNM	American College of Nurse-Midwives
ACP	American College of Physicians
ACR	American College of Radiology
ACS	American College of Surgeons
ACTA	American Cardiovascular Technologists Association
ACTA	American Corrective Therapy Association
ADA	American Dental Association
ADA	American Dietetic Association
ADAA	American Dental Assistants Association
ADHA	American Dental Hygienists' Association
ADTA	American Dance Therapy Association
AES	American Electroencephalographic Society
AHA	American Hospital Association
AHCPR	Agency for Health Care Policy and Research (now AHRQ)
AHPA	American Health Planning Association

Chart continued on following page

Abbreviatons for Selected Health Care Organizations, Associations, and Agencies
Continued

AHRQ	Agency for Healthcare Research and Quality
AIBS	American Institute of Biological Sciences
AIHA	American Industrial Hygiene Association
AIUM	American Institute of Ultrasound in Medicine
AMA	American Medical Association
AMEA	American Medical Electroencephalographic Association
AMI	Association of Medical Illustrators
AMIA	American Medical Informatics Association
AmSECT	American Society of Extra-Corporeal Technology
AMSN	Academy of Medical-Surgical Nurses
AMT	American Medical Technologists
ANA	American Nurses Association
ANCC	American Nurses Credentialing Center
ANF	American Nurses Foundation
ANHA	American Nursing Homes Association
ANNA	American Nephrology Nurses' Association
ANRC	American National Red Cross
AOA	American Optometric Association
AOA	American Osteopathic Association
AONE	American Organization of Nurse Executives
AORN	Association of Operating Room Nurses
AOTA	American Occupational Therapy Association
APA	American Podiatry Association
APA	American Psychiatric Association
APA	American Psychological Association

**Abbreviations for Selected Health Care
Organizations, Associations, and Agencies**
Continued

APAP	Association of Physician Assistants Programs
APHA	American Public Health Association
APIC	Association of Practitioners in Infection Control
APTA	American Physical Therapy Association
ARCA	American Rehabilitation Counseling Association
ARN	Association of Rehabilitation Nurses
ASA	American Society of Anesthesiologists
ASAHP	American Society of Allied Health Professionals
ASC	American Society of Cytotechnology
ASCO	American Society of Clinical Oncology
ASCP	American Society of Clinical Pathologists
ASE	American Society of Echocardiography
ASET	American Society of Electroencephalographic Technologists
ASHA	American Speech and Hearing Association
ASIA	American Spinal Injury Association
ASIM	American Society of Internal Medicine
ASM	American Society of Microbiology
ASMT	American Society for Medical Technology
ASNSA	American Society of Nursing Service Administrators
ASPAN	American Association of Post Anesthesia Nurses
ASPH	Association of Schools of Public Health

Chart continued on following page

Abbreviatons for Selected Health Care Organizations, Associations, and Agencies
Continued

ASRT	American Society of Radiologic Technologists
AST	Association of Surgical Technologists
ASTRO	American Society of Therapeutic Radiation Oncology
ASUTS	American Society of Ultrasound Technical Specialists
ATS	American Thoracic Society
AUPHA	Association of University Programs in Health Administration
AVA	American Vocational Association
AVMA	American Veterinary Medical Association
CAHEA (AMA)	Committee on Allied Health Education and Accreditation
CAP	College of American Pathologists
CCHFA	Canadian Council of Health Facilities Accreditation
CCHSE	Canadian Council of Health Service Executives
CCNE	Commission on Collegiate Nursing Education
CDC	Centers for Disease Control and Prevention
CGFNS	Commission on Graduates of Foreign Nursing Schools
CGNA	Canadian Gerontological Nursing Association
CME (AMA)	Council on Medical Education of the American Medical Association
CNA	Canadian Nurses Association
COEAMRA	Council on Education of the American Medical Record Association
DHHS	Department of Health and Human Services
ENA	Emergency Nurses Association

**Abbreviations for Selected Health Care
Organizations, Associations, and Agencies**
Continued

FDA	Food and Drug Administration
HCFA	Health Care Financing Administration
HRA	Health Resources Administration
HSCA	Health Sciences Communications Association
HSRA	Health Services and Resources Administration
IAET	International Association for Enterostomal Therapy
IOM	Institute of Medicine of the National Academy of Sciences
ISCV	International Society for Cardiovascular surgery
JCAHO	Joint Commission on the Accreditation of Healthcare Organizations
JCAHPO	Joint Commission on Allied Health Personnel in Ophthalmology
MLA	Medical Library Association
NAACLS	National Accrediting Agency for Clinical Laboratory Science
NAACOG	Nurses Association of the American College of Obstetrics and Gynecology
NACA	National Advisory Council on Aging-Canadian
NACCHO	National Association of County and City Health Officials
NACT	National Alliance of Cardiovascular Technologists
NADONA/LTC	National Association of Directors of Nursing Administration in Long Term Care
NAEMT	National Association of Emergency Medical Technicians

Chart continued on following page

Abbreviatons for Selected Health Care Organizations, Associations, and Agencies
Continued

NAHC	National Association of Home Care
NAHSR	National Association of Human Services Technologists
NAMT	National Association for Music Therapy
NANDA	North American Nursing Diagnosis Association
NANT	National Association of Nephrology Technologists
NAPNES	National Association for Practical Nurse Education and Services
NARF	National Association of Rehabilitation Facilities
NASMD	National Association of State Medical Directors
NASW	National Association of Social Workers
NATTS	National Association of Trade and Technical Schools
NBNA	National Black Nurses Association
NCEHPHP	National Council on the Education of Health Professionals in Health Promotion
NCHS	National Center for Health Statistics
NCRE	National Council on Rehabilitation Education
NEHA	National Environmental Health Association
NFLPN	National Federation of Licensed Practical Nurses
NHC	National Health Council
NHSC	National Health Services Corps
NIH	National Institutes of Health
NIOSH	National Institute of Occupational Safety and Health
NKF	National Kidney Foundation
NLN	National League for Nursing

**Abbreviations for Selected Health Care
Organizations, Associations, and Agencies**
Continued

NNBA	National Nurses in Business Association
NOLF	Nursing Organization Liaison Forum
NONPF	National Organization of Nurse Practitioner Faculties
NPWH	National Association of Nurse Practitioners in Women's Health
NRCA	National Rehabilitation Counseling Association
NREMT	National Registry of Emergency Medical Technicians
NSCPT	National Society for Cardiopulmonary Technology
NSH	National Society for Histotechnology
NSNA	National Student Nurses Association
NTRS	National Therapeutic Recreation Society
NTSAD	National Tay-Sachs and Allied Diseases Association
OAA	Opticians Association of America
ONS	Oncology Nurses Association
PNAA	Philippine Nurses Association of America
RWJF	The Robert Wood Johnson Foundation
SAAABB	Subcommittee on Accreditation of the American Association of Blood Banks
SDMS	Society of Diagnostic Medical Sonographers
SNIVT	Society of Non-invasive Vascular Technology
SNM	Society of Nuclear Medicine
SNM-TS	Society of Nuclear Medicine-Technologists Section

Chart continued on following page

**Abbreviatons for Selected Health Care
Organizations, Associations, and Agencies**
Continued

SOPHE	Society for Public Health Education
STS	Society of Thoracic Surgeons
STTI	Sigma Theta Tau International
SVS	Society for Vascular Surgery
TAANA	The American Association of Nurse Attorneys
USPHS	United States Public Health Service
VA	Veterans Affairs
WHO	World Health Organization

Professional Designations for Health Care Providers*

Degrees, certifications, memberships and other initials that precede or follow the names of health care providers often provide helpful information regarding their area of expertise and level of practice. The following list identifies commonly used designations in English-speaking countries.

ACSW	Academy of Certified Social Workers
AN	Associate Nurse
ANP	Adult Nurse Practitioner
APRN, BC	Advanced Practice Registered Nurse, Board Certified
ARNP	Advanced Registered Nurse Practitioner
ARRT	American Registry of Radiologic Technologists
BA	Bachelor of Arts
BB(ASCP)	Technologist in Blood Banking certified by The American Society of Clinical Pathologists
BDentSci	Bachelor of Dental Science
BDS	Bachelor of Dental Surgery
BDSc	Bachelor of Dental Science
BHS	Bachelor of Health Science
BHyg	Bachelor of Hygiene
BM	Bachelor of Medicine
BMed	Bachelor of Medicine
BMedBiol	Bachelor of Medical Biology
BMedSci	Bachelor of Medical Science
BMic	Bachelor of Microbiology

Chart continued on following page

---

*From Miller-Keane: Encyclopedia & Dictionary of Medicine, Nursing, & Allied Health, 7th ed. Philadelphia, WB Saunders, 2003.

Professional Designations for Health Care Providers *Continued*

BMS	Bachelor of Medical Science
BMT	Bachelor of Medical Technology
BO	Bachelor of Osteopathy
BP	Bachelor of Pharmacy
BPH	Bachelor of Public Health
BPharm	Bachelor of Pharmacy
BPHEng	Bachelor of Public Health Engineering
BPHN	Bachelor of Public Health Nursing
BPsTh	Bachelor of Psychotherapy
BS	Bachelor of Science
BSM	Bachelor of Science in Medicine
BSN	Bachelor of Science in Nursing
BSPh	Bachelor of Science in Pharmacy
BSS	Bachelor of Sanitary Science
BVMS	Bachelor of Veterinary Medicine and Science
BVSc	Bachelor of Veterinary Science
CAC	Certified Alcohol Counselor
CALN	Clinical Administrative Liaison Nurse
CANP	Certified Adult Nurse Practitioner
C(ASCP)	Technologist in Chemistry certified by the American Society of Clinical Pathologists
CB	Bachelor of Surgery
CCRN	Critical Care Registered Nurse
CCT	Certified Cardiographic Technician
CDA	Certified Dental Assistant
CDC	Certified Drug Counselor
CEN	Certificate for Emergency Nursing
CEO	Chief Executive Officer
CFNP	Certified Family Nurse Practitioner
ChB	Bachelor of Surgery
ChD	Doctor of Surgery
CHES	Certified Health Education Specialist
ChM	Master of Surgery

Professional Designations for Health Care Providers *Continued*

CIC	Certified in Infection Control
CIH	Certificate in Industrial Health
CLA	Certified Laboratory Assistant
CLS	Clinical Laboratory Scientist
CLS(NCA)	Clinical Laboratory Scientist certified by the National Certification Agency for Medical Laboratory Personnel
CLT	Certified Laboratory Technician; Clinical Laboratory Technician
CLT(NCA)	Laboratory Technician certified by the National Certification Agency for Medical Laboratory Personnel
CM	Master of Surgery
CMA	Certified Medical Assistant
CMO	Chief Medical Officer
CMT	Chief Medical Transcriptionist
CNA	Certified Nursing Assistant
CNM	Certified Nurse-Midwife
CNMT	Certified Nuclear Medicine Technologist
CNOR	Certified Nurse, Operating Room
CNP	Community Nurse Practitioner
CNS	Clinical Nurse Specialist
CORN	Certified Operating Room Nurse
CORT	Certified Operating Room Technician
COTA	Certified Occupational Therapy Assistant
CPAN	Certified Post Anesthesia Nurse
CPH	Certified in Public Health
CPNP	Certified Pediatric Nurse Practitioner
CPTA	Certified Physical Therapy Assistant
CRNA	Certified Registered Nurse Anesthetist
CRNP	Certified Registered Nurse Practitioner

Chart continued on following page

Professional Designations for Health Care Providers *Continued*

CRRN	Certified Registered Rehabilitation Nurse
CRRT	Certified Registered Respiratory Therapist
CRTT	Certified Respiratory Therapy Technician
CSN	Certified School Nurse
CT(ASCP)	Cytotechnologist certified by the American Society of Clinical Pathologists
CURN	Certified Urological Registered Nurse
CVO	Chief Veterinary Officer
DA	Dental Assistant; Diploma in Anesthetics
DC	Doctor of Chiropractic
DCH	Diploma in Child Health
DCh	Doctor of Surgery
DChO	Doctor of Ophthalmic Surgery
DCM	Doctor of Comparative Medicine
DCOG	Diploma of the College of Obstetricians and Gynaecologists
DCP	Diploma in Clinical Pathology; Diploma in Clinical Psychology
DDH	Diploma in Dental Health
DDM	Doctor of Dental Medicine; Diploma in Dermatologic Medicine DDO Diploma in Dental Orthopaedics
DDR	Diploma in Dental Radiology
DDS	Doctor of Dental Surgery
DDSc	Doctor of Dental Science
DFHom	Diploma in the Faculty of Homeopathy
DHg	Doctor of Hygiene
DHy	Doctor of Hygiene
DHyg	Doctor of Hygiene
Dip	Diplomate
DipBact	Diploma in Bacteriology
DipChern	Diploma in Chemistry

Professional Designations for Health Care Providers *Continued*

DipClinPath	Diploma in Clinical Pathology
DipMicrobiol	Diploma in Microbiology
DipSocMed	Diploma in Social Medicine
DLM(ASCP)	Diplomate in Laboratory Management
DMD	Doctor of Dental Medicine
DMT	Doctor of Medical Technology
DMV	Doctor of Veterinary Medicine
DN	Doctor of Nursing
DNE	Doctor of Nursing Education
DNS	Doctor of Nursing Science
DNSc	Doctor of Nursing Science
DO	Doctor of Ophthalmology; Doctor of Optometry; Doctor of Osteopathy
DON	Doctor of Nursing
DOS	Doctor of Ocular Science; Doctor of Optical Science
DP	Doctor of Pharmacy; Doctor of Podiatry
DHP	Doctor of Public Health; Doctor of Public Hygiene
DPhC	Doctor of Pharmaceutical Chemistry
DPHN	Doctor of Public Health Nursing
DPhys	Diploma in Physiotherapy
DPM	Doctor of Physical Medicine; Doctor of Podiatric Medicine; Doctor of Preventive Medicine; Doctor of Psychiatric Medicine
Dr	Doctor
DrHyg	Doctor of Hygiene
DrMed	Doctor of Medicine
DrPH	Doctor of Public Health; Doctor of Public Hygiene
DSc	Doctor of Science
DSE	Doctor of Sanitary Engineering
DSIM	Doctor of Science in Industrial Medicine
DSSc	Diploma in Sanitary Science

Chart continued on following page

**Professional Designations for Health Care
Providers** *Continued*

DVM	Doctor of Veterinary Medicine
DVMS	Doctor of Veterinary Medicine and Surgery
DVR	Doctor of Veterinary Radiology
DVS	Doctor of Veterinary Science; Doctor of Veterinary Medicine DVSc Doctor of Veterinary Science
EdD	Doctor of Education
EMT	Emergency Medical Technician
EMT-P	Emergency Medical Technician–Paramedic
ET	Enterostornal Therapist
FAAN	Fellow of the American Academy of Nurses
FACA	Fellow of the American College of Anesthetists; Fellow of the American College of Angiology; Fellow of the American College of Apothecaries
FACAI	Fellow of the American College of Allergists
FACC	Fellow of the American College of Cardiologists
FACCP	Fellow of the American College of Chest Physicians
FACD	Fellow of the American College of Dentists
FACFP	Fellow of the American College of family Physicians
FACG	Fellow of the American College of Gastroenterology
FACHA	Fellow of the American College of Health Administrators
FACOG	Fellow of the American College of Obstetricians and Gynecologists
FACP	Fellow of the American College of Physicians
FACPM	Fellow of the American College of Preventive Medicine

Professional Designations for Health Care Providers *Continued*

FACS	Fellow of the American College of Surgeons
FACSM	Fellow of the American College of Sports Medicine
FAMA	Fellow of the American Medical Association
FAOTA	Fellow of the American Occupational Therapy Association
FAPA	Fellow of the American Psychiatric Association
FAPHA	Fellow of the American Public Health Association
FBPsS	Fellow of the British Psychological Society
FCAP	Fellow of the College of American Pathologists
FCMS	Fellow of the College of Medicine and Surgery
FCO	Fellow of the College of Osteopathy
FCPS	Fellow of the College of Physicians and Surgeons
FCSP	Fellow of the Chartered Society of Physiotherapy
FCST	Fellow of the College of Speech Therapists
FDS	Fellow in Dental Surgery
FDSRCSEng	Fellow in Dental Surgery of the Royal College of Surgeons of England
FFA	Fellow of the Faculty of Anesthetists
FFCM	Fellow of the Faculty of Community Medicine
FFD	Fellow of the Faculty of Dentistry
FFOM	Fellow of the Faculty of Occupational Medicine
FFR	Fellow of the Faculty of Radiologists
FIB	Fellow in the Institute of Biology

Chart continued on following page

Professional Designations for Health Care Providers *Continued*

FICD	Fellow of the Institute of Canadian Dentists; Fellow of the International College of Dentists
FIMLT	Fellow of Institute of Medical Laboratory Technology
FNP	Family Nurse Practitioner
FPS	Fellow of the Pathological Society
FRCD	Fellow of the Royal College of Dentists
FRCGP	Fellow of the Royal College of General Practitioners
FRCOG	Fellow of the Royal College of Obstetricians and Gynaecologists
FRCP	Fellow of the Royal College of Physicians
FRCPath	Fellow of the Royal College of Pathologists
FRCP(C)	Fellow of the Royal College of Physicians of Canada
FRCS	Fellow of the Royal College of Surgeons
FRCS(C)	Fellow of the Royal College of Surgeons of Canada
GNP	Gerontological Nurse Practitioner
H(ASCP)	Technologist in Hematology certified by the American Society of Clinical Pathologists
HT(ASCP)	Histologic Technician certified by the American Society of Clinical Pathologists
HTL(ASCP)	Histotechnologist certified by the American Society of Clinical Pathologists
I(ASCP)	Technologist in Immunology certified by the American Society of Clinical Pathologists
LCSW	Licensed Clinical Social Worker
LMCC	Licentiate of the Medical Council of Canada

Professional Designations for Health Care Providers *Continued*

LMRCP	Licentiate in Midwifery of the Royal College of Physicians
LOT	Licensed Occupational Therapist
LPN	Licensed Practical Nurse
LPT	Licensed Physical Therapist
LVN	Licensed Vocational Nurse
MA	Master of Arts
M(ASCP)	Technologist in Microbiology certified by the American Society of Clinical Pathologists
MB	Bachelor of Medicine
MC	Master of Surgery
MCIS	Master of Computer and Information Science; Master of Computer Information Systems
MCPS	Member of the College of Physicians and Surgeons
MD	Doctor of Medicine
MDentSc	Master of Dental Science
MDS	Master of Dental Surgery
MHA	Master in Healthcare Administration
MHC	Mental Health Counselor
MLT	Medical Laboratory Technician
MLT(ASCP)	Medical Laboratory Technician certified by the American Society of Clinical Pathologists
MMS	Master of Medical Science
MMSA	Master of Midwifery
MPH	Master of Public Health
MPharm	Master of Pharmacy
MRad	Master of Radiology
MRL	Medical Records Librarian
MS	Master of Science; Master of Surgery
MSB	Master of Science in Bacteriology
MSc	Master of Science
MScD	Master of Dental Science

Chart continued on following page

Professional Designations for Health Care Providers *Continued*

MScN	Master of Science in Nursing
MSN	Master of Science in Nursing
MSPH	Master of Science in Public Health
MSPhar	Master of Science in Pharmacy
MSSc	Master of Sanitary Science
MSW	Master of Social Work; Medical Social Worker
MT	Medical Technologist
MT(ASCP)	Medical Technologist certified by the American Society of Clinical Pathologists
MVD	Doctor of Veterinary Medicine
NA	Nurses Aide
ND	Doctor of Nursing
NHA	Nursing Home Administrator
NM(ASCP)	Technologist in Nuclear Medicine certified by the American Society of Clinical Pathologists
NMT	Nuclear Medicine Technologist
NNP	Neonatal Nurse Practitioner
NP	Nurse Practitioner
OD	Doctor of Optometry
ONC	Orthopedic Nursing Certificate
ORT	Operating Room Technician
OT	Occupational Therapist
OTL	Occupational Therapist, Licensed
OTR	Occupational Therapist, Registered
OTReg	Occupational Therapist, Registered
PA	Physician's Assistant
PA-C	Physician Assistant - Certified
PBT(ASCP)	Phlebotomy Technician certified by the American Society of Clinical Pathologists
PCP	Primary Care Physician
PD	Doctor of Pharmacy
PharmD	Doctor of Pharmacy
PhD	Doctor of Philosophy; Doctor of Pharmacy

Professional Designations for Health Care Providers *Continued*

PHN	Public Health Nurse
PNP	Pediatric Nurse Practitioner
PT	Physical Therapist
PTA	Physical Therapy Assistant
RDA	Registered Dental Assistant
RDMS	Registered Diagnostic Medical Sonographer
REEGT	Registered Electroencephalogram Technologist
Reg	Registered
RHIA	Registered Health Information Administrator
RHIT	Registered Health Information Technician
RMA	Registered Medical Assistant
RN	Registered Nurse
RNA	Registered Nurse Anesthetist
RN, BC	Registered Nurse, Board Certified
RN, C	Registered Nurse, Certified
RN, CNA	Registered Nurse, Certified in Nursing Administration
RN, CNAA	Registered Nurse, Certified in Nursing Administration, Advanced
RN, CNA, BC	Registered Nurse, Certified in Nursing Administration, Board Certified
RN, CS	Registered Nurse, Certified Specialist
RPh	Registered Pharmacist
RPT	Registered Physical Therapist
RPTA	Registered Physical Therapist Assistant
RRL	Registered Record Librarian
RRT	Registered Respiratory Therapist
RT	Radiologic Technologist; Respiratory Therapist
RT(N)	Nuclear Medicine Technologist

Chart continued on following page

Professional Designations for Health Care Providers *Continued*

RT(R)	Technologist in Diagnostic Radiology
RTR	Registered Recreational Therapist
RT(T)	Radiation Therapy Technologist
SBB(ASCP)	Specialist in Blood Banking certified by the American Society of Clinical Pathologists
ScD	Doctor of Science
SCT(ASCP)	Specialist in Cytotechnology certified by the American Society of Clinical Pathologists
SLP	Speech and Language Pathologist
SNP	School Nurse Practitioner
ST	Speech Therapist; Surgical Technologist
SW	Social Worker

Surgical Terminology and Technology*

The following terms are commonly used in surgery and anesthesia. They include terms related to surgical and anesthetic instrumentation and procedures.

Term	Definition
ablation	removal by erosion or vaporization, usually due to intense heat
abscess	a localized area of pus in the body
absorbable suture	any suture that is digested by body tissue
ampule	a small glass container that holds medication that has been sterilized
analgesia	the absence of pain
anastomosis	the surgical formation of a passageway between two spaces, hollow organs, or lumens
anesthetic	an agent that produces analgesia
appose	to bring two structures together
approximate	to bring body parts or tissues together by sutures or other means
armboard	detachable extension on the operating table that accommodates the patient's arms

Chart continued on following page

---

*Modified from Fuller J: Surgical technology, 3rd ed. Philadelphia, WB Saunders, 1993.

Surgical Terminology and Technology
Continued

Term	Definition
aspirate	to withdraw fluids or gases by means of suction, as when removing fluid from the body with a syringe; also refers to the material thus obtained
atraumatic	refers to a suture-needle combination that has no needle eye; the suture is swaged into the end of the needle shaft
autoclave	steam sterilizer
autotransfusion	transfusion using the patient's own blood
Bankart procedure	operation of the shoulder girdle to treat recurrent shoulder dislocation
bifurcated	Y-shaped; divided into two branches
biopsy	removal of a small piece of tissue from a living body for microscopic examination
bipolar	refers to a type of electrosurgical unit in which the electrical current is localized at the tip of the electrocautery probe and does not pass through the patient
bipolar coagulation	electrosurgery that utilizes forceps rather than an electrosurgical pencil
bleeder	a severed blood vessel
blunt dissection	the separation of tissues or tissue planes with an instrument that has no cutting ability

Surgical Terminology and Technology
Continued

Term	Definition
bolsters	tubing through which retention sutures are threaded to prevent them from cutting into the patient's skin
bone wax	medical-grade beeswax used on bone tissue to control bleeding
Bovie cleaner	small, rough-surfaced pad used to clean the electrocautery tip during surgery
box lock	the ratchet closure mechanism of many surgical instruments
Brown & Sharp (B&S) gauge	sizing standard used to measure steel sutures
bur	a round instrument with sharp cutting edges used for drilling holes in bone
calipers	an instrument with two bent or curved legs used for measuring thickness or diameter of a solid
caudal anesthetic	an anesthetic agent introduced into the caudal canal to induce a type of epidural anesthesia
chromic salts	chemicals used to treat surgical gut suture so that it resists digestion by body tissues
circulator	surgical team member who does not perform a surgical hand scrub or don sterile attire and thus does not work within the sterile field

Chart continued on following page

Surgical Terminology and Technology
Continued

Term	Definition
clamp	instrument designed to hold tissue, objects (such as surgical needles), or fabric (such as a towel)
cleaning	a process that removes organic or inorganic debris
closed anesthesia system	in general anesthesia, the recirculation of anesthetic gases through the gas machine and back to the patient that prevents exposure of personnel to the gases
closed gloving	method of donning sterile gloves when a surgical gown is worn
closed reduction	a process in which bone fragments are reduced manually, without surgical intervention
coagulation	clotting of blood
communicate	to connect; used to describe the relationship between two structures or organs that connect
curette	a spoon-shaped instrument used to scrape tissue from a surface
cutting instrument	any instrument with a sharp edge
dead space	an area lying between tissue layers or opposing them that the surgeon has not approximated; dead space within a wound can lead to infection
debridement	a process of removing dead skin, debris, or foreign bodies from a wound

Surgical Terminology and Technology
Continued

Term	Definition
defibrillator	a piece of equipment used to generate electrical impulses to the heart during cardiac arrest in an attempt to restart the heartbeat
deflect	to peel or retract back and away but not detach
dehiscence	the splitting apart of a surgical wound after surgery
dermabrasion	the physical sanding of the skin to remove pockmarks and other scars
desiccation	the drying up of a substance
dilators	graduated, rodlike instruments used to enlarge the diameter of a channel or duct
dissector	a tiny sponge mounted on a clamp and used to perform blunt dissection
divide	to cut or sever
dorsal recumbent	position of the patient lying on his or her back; synonymous with *supine*
drill bit	in orthopedics, an instrument used in a drill to create a hole in bone to accommodate a screw
emergence	the arousal from general anesthesia after cessation of the anesthetic agent

Chart continued on following page

Surgical Terminology and Technology
Continued

Term	Definition
endotracheal tube	tube that is inserted into the patient's trachea for the administration of anesthetic gas
endotracheal tube fire	a fire that occurs within the patient's endotracheal tube during laser surgery that causes immediate and severe trauma to the lungs
epidural	type of anesthetic agent that is introduced into the epidural space of the spine
Esmarch bandage	rolled rubber bandage that is wrapped around the limb to force blood away from the surgical site before the application of a tourniquet
ethylene oxide gas	highly flammable, toxic gas that is capable of sterilizing an object
evisceration	in surgery, the splitting open of a surgical wound and subsequent spillage of its contents
excise	to remove by cutting out
excitement	the second stage of general anesthesia in which the patient is sensitive to external stimuli
exposure	the anatomic area that the surgeon can see and thus operate on
extractor	in orthopedics, an instrument used to remove a metal implant from bone
fiberoptic	a flexible material that carries light along its length; refers to the fibers of glass or plastic that are

Surgical Terminology and Technology
Continued

Term	Definition
	bundled together to form the cables used for endoscopic examination
first intention	a process by which a clean surgical wound heals directly, without granulation
fistula	an abnormal passageway from a normal cavity to the outside of the body or another cavity
fixation	in orthopedics, to hold bone fragments in place following a fracture; in *external* fixation, the fragments are held in alignment by an external device, such as a plaster cast; in *internal* fixation, fragments are held in alignment with an appliance such as a rod, nail, or screw
flaking	the tendency of some suture materials to release tiny particles of the suture in the wound
flash autoclave	an autoclave used in surgery to sterilize equipment quickly by steam under pressure
footboard	section of the operating table at the foot end that can be removed or angled up or down
four-by-four (4 × 4)	type of surgical sponge consisting of loosely woven gauze squares
Fowler position	sitting position
fracture	the breaking of a part of the body, especially bone; different

Chart continued on following page

Surgical Terminology and Technology
Continued

Term	Definition
fracture *continued*	types of fractures include: (1) *comminuted*—the bone is splintered into many small fragments; (2) *compound*—the fracture penetrates adjacent soft tissue and skin (also called an *open* fracture); (3) *greenstick—the fracture* extends only partially through the bone; incomplete; commonly occurs in children; (4) *impacted*—a portion of the bone is traumatically driven into another bone or fragment; (5) *pathologic*—caused by disease rather than injury; (6) *spiral*—the fracture forms a spiral pattern; the bone has been twisted apart; (7) *transverse*—the fracture line lies perpendicular to the long axis of the bone
free tie	a term used by the surgeon when he or she requests a length of suture for ligation
French-eye	a delicate needle whose eye contains a spring
friable	refers to any tissue that is easily torn
frozen section	a fine slice of frozen biopsy tissue that is microscopically examined for the presence of disease
full length	refers to the length of a suture strand; full length is 54 or 60 inches
gauge	in orthopedics, an instrument used to measure the depth of a hole made by a drill bit

Surgical Terminology and Technology
Continued

Term	Definition
Gelfoam	medical-grade gelatin that is used to control capillary bleeding
general anesthetic	type of anesthetic agent that causes unconsciousness
glutaraldehyde	chemical capable of rendering objects sterile
gouge	in orthopedic surgery, an instrument used to create a grooved surface on bone
gravity displacement sterilizer	type of sterilizer that removes air by gravity
grounding cable	during electrosurgery, the cable connecting the control unit to the inactive electrode
grounding pad	gel-covered pad that grounds the patient during electrosurgery; inactive electrode
gurney	stretcher
headboard	removable section of the operating table at the head end that can be angled up or down
hemostasis	the control of hemorrhage during surgery
hemostat	an instrument used to clamp a blood vessel
hemostatic agent	a drug that promotes blood coagulation

Chart continued on following page

Surgical Terminology and Technology
Continued

Term	Definition
high vacuum sterilizer	type of steam sterilizer that removes air in the chamber by vacuum
impactor	in orthopedics, an instrument used to drive an implant into bone; may also be called a *driver*
incise	to cut or sever with a cutting instrument
induction	the first stage of general anesthesia during which the patient's physiologic status is unstable
inflammation	the localized, protective reaction of tissue to injury or disease
infusion pump	containment and **monitoring** equipment used when the patient receives intravenous solutions, including anesthetics
intentional hypotension	during surgery, the intentional lowering of a patient's blood pressure to control hemorrhage
intentional hypothermia	during surgery, the intentional lowering of a patient's core temperature to control hemorrhage
Javid shunt	a commercially prepared length of plastic tubing used to bypass the carotid artery temporarily during carotid endarterectomy
jaws	the working end of a surgical instrument
Kerlix bandage	a rolled bandage made of soft, woven material

Surgical Terminology and Technology
Continued

Term	Definition
Kraske position	operative position used for procedure of the perianal area; the patient lies in prone position, with the table broken at its midsection so that the head and feet are lower than the midsection; also called *jackknife* position or *knee-chest* position
laminectomy position	operative position used for spinal surgery; a form of the prone position
laparotomy tape	the largest surgical sponge available, used during major surgery; also called a *lap tape*
laser	acronym for **l**ight **a**mplification by **s**timulated **e**mission of **r**adiation; a device that generates a beam of extremely bright light of a single color
ligate	to tie a length of suture around a vessel or duct and secure it with knots
ligation clips	small V-shaped clips that are applied around blood vessels or ducts in place of a ligature; sometimes referred to as *silver clips*
local anesthetic	type of anesthetic agent that causes loss of sensation or feeling in a localized area
local infiltration	procedure in which the anesthetic is injected directly into the operative tissue

Chart continued on following page

Surgical Terminology and Technology
Continued

Term	Definition
lumen	hollow tube
microfibrillar collagen hemostat	a substance derived from collagen and used as a hemostatic agent
monitored anesthesia care	procedure in which the patient receives an intravenous sedative anesthetic which may be given in conjunction with a local anesthetic or by itself
monofilament suture	suture composed of a single, nonfibrous strand of material
monopolar	refers to a type of electrosurgical unit in which the electrical current passes through the patient and back to the control unit
multifilament suture	suture composed of many fine strands of fiber that are twisted or braided together
nail	orthopedic device used to fasten together pieces of bone; examples are Neufeld nail, Jewett nail, Ken sliding nail, and Smith-Petersen nail
nerve block	anesthesia of a large single nerve or nerves
neuromuscular blocking agent	a pharmaceutical agent that causes paralysis during general anesthesia
nonabsorbable suture	suture that is never digested by tissue but becomes encapsulated by it

Surgical Terminology and Technology
Continued

Term	Definition
open gloving	method of donning sterile surgical gloves when a gown is not worn
open reduction	to reduce bone fragments with surgical instruments
orthopedic cutdown instruments	instruments used to gain access to fractures or to operate on soft tissue injuries; includes scalpel handles, tissue forceps, Metzenbaum scissors, Mayo scissors, needle holders, mosquito clamps, Allis clamps, Kelly clamps, Kocher clamps, and Mayo clamps
orthopedic cutting instruments	instruments used to cut bone; examples are *rasps* (to smooth the surface of a bone or remove the medullary cavity so a stemmed prosthesis can be inserted), *reamers* (used to form hollow area in the bone), *knives* (to cut away heavy connective tissue such as cartilage), *elevators* (used to lift the periosteum from the surface of the bone or to perform fine dissection during tendon and ligament repair), *ronqeurs* (used to cut bone), *saws* (power-driven and used to cut through fine bone), *osteotomes* (to create slivers of bone used in a graft), *curette* (used to spoon out bits of bone from a curved area), *gouge*

Chart continued on following page

Surgical Terminology and Technology
Continued

Term	Definition
orthopedic cutting instruments *continued*	(used to create a grooved surface on the bone), and *drills* (used in conjunction with a drill bit to drill a hole)
orthopedic internal fiixation devices	surgical steel or alloy appliances used to stabilize a fracture during healing; examples are pins and bolts, nails, plates, staples, and screws
orthopedic measuring devices	instruments used in implant procedures; examples are *calipers* (used to measure the width of a ball joint head in preparation for a prosthetic implant) and *depth gauges* (used to measure the depth of the hole made by a drill to determine what length of screw is needed)
osteotome	a chisel-like instrument used with a mallet to cut bone
oxidized cellulose	medical-grade cellulose manufactured into mesh squares and used as a hemostatic agent
PACU	acronym for postanesthesia care unit
patty	a type of sponge used during neurosurgery
peracetic acid	chemical capable of rendering objects sterile
pin	device used in orthopedics to fasten together pieces of bone; pins are inserted with a drill or driver; examples are Steinmann pin and Knowles pin; also used

Surgical Terminology and Technology
Continued

Term	Definition
	as a verb, meaning to secure and immobilize fragments of bone
plate	orthopedic flat internal fixation device held in place with screws; examples are adjustable McLaughlin plate, Moe intertrochanteric plate, and Bagby compression plate
points	the tips of a surgical instrument
probe	an instrument placed within a lumen to determine its length and direction
prosthesis	any artificial organ or body part
pursestring	a technique of suturing; a continuous strand is passed in and out around the circumference of a hollow structure and then is pulled tight like a drawstring
rachets	interlocking clasps that hold a finger ring instrument closed
reamer	an instrument used in orthopedic surgery to create a hollow area in bone
reduce	in orthopedics, to bring two bone fragments in alignment after a fracture
reel	a continuous strand of suture mounted on a spool; used for ligation of many blood vessels in rapid succession

Chart continued on following page

Surgical Terminology and Technology
Continued

Term	Definition
resect	to cut out and remove a section of tissue
retention suture	heavy, nonabsorbable sutures placed behind the skin sutures and underneath all tissue layers to give added strength to the closure
retract	to pull tissues back or away to expose a structure or other tissue
reverse Trendelenburg position	operative position in which the patient lies in supine position and the operating table is tilted so that the head is higher than the feet
running suture	a method of suturing that uses one continuous suture that is passed over and under the tissue edges
self-tapping	in orthopedics, a screw that creates its own hole in bone as it is being inserted
shank	the area of a surgical instrument between the box lock and the finger ring
sharp dissection	the use of a scalpel or other sharp instrument for the separation of tissues
shelf life	the amount of time a wrapped object will remain sterile after it has been subjected to a sterilization process

Surgical Terminology and Technology
Continued

Term	Definition
Sims position	position of the patient lying on his or her side; also called *lateral* position
sizer	a dummy or model of a prosthesis used to determine the correct size of prosthesis needed during an operation
specimen	any tissue, foreign body, prosthesis, or fluid that is removed from the patient
speculum	an instrument used for exposure of a body cavity, such as the nose
sponge stick	a folded four-by-four mounted on a sponge clamp
steam sterilizer	sterilizer that exposes objects to high-pressure steam
sterile	completely free of living microorganisms
sterile field	an area that encompasses draped equipment, scrubbed personnel, and the draped patient
stick tie	name given to suture ligature—a suture-needle combination that is passed through a vessel or duct before ligation to prevent it from slipping off the edge of the structure
surgeon's preference card	file card that contains information pertaining to suture materials, equipment, or special instruments used by a particular surgeon

Chart continued on following page

Surgical Terminology and Technology
Continued

Term	Definition
surgical drape	sterile cloth or nonwoven material placed around the surgical site to create a sterile field
surgical scrub	precise method by which all team members who will be working in sterile attire scrub their hands and arms before performing an operation
surgically clean	as clean as possible without being sterile
suture	a material used to bring tissues together by sewing; can also refer to a suture-needle combination
suture ligature	a needle-suture combination used to tie a bleeding vessel and attach it to nearby tissue simultaneously, thus preventing the tie from slipping off the end of the vessel
table breaks	hinged sections of the operating table that can be folded up or down to create different postures
tenaculum	an instrument used to grasp tissue
tensile strength	the amount of stress a suture will withstand before breaking
terminal disinfection	a process in which an area or object is rendered disinfected after contamination has occurred

Surgical Terminology and Technology
Continued

Term	Definition
tie-on passer	a strand of suture material whose end is secured to the end of a long clamp; used to ligate deep vessels where exposure is limited
topical anesthetic	a drug used on the surface of tissue, such as the eye
topical thrombin	drug used in conjunction with gelatin sponges to halt capillary bleeding
torsion	the twisting of an organ or structure upon itself that often causes diminished blood supply to the affected area
tourniquet	a device that prevents the flow of blood to the surgical wound
transect	to cut across an organ or section of tissue
Trendelenburg position	operative position in which the patient lies in supine position with the operating table tilted so that the head is lower than the feet
trocar	a spear-shaped instrument or needle
Webril	a soft, rolled cotton material used to pad a limb before the application of a plaster cast

Classes of Drugs and Their Uses

This is an alphabetized list of drugs with brand name in parentheses and explanation of use (class or type).

Generic (Brand Name)	Explanation of Use
acarbose (Precose)	Antidiabetic/type 2/ alphaglucoside inhibitor
acetaminophen (Tylenol)	Analgesic/mild
acyclovir (Zovirax)	Antiviral
albuterol (Proventil)	Bronchodilator
alendronate (Fosamax)	Antiosteoporosis/ bisphosphonate
alprazolam (Xanax)	Tranquilizer/minor/ benzodiazepine
aluminum antacid (Rolaids)	GI/antacid
aluminum+ magnesium antacid (Gaviscon)	GI/antacid
amiodarone (Cordarone)	Cardiovascular/antiarrhythmic
amlodipine (Norvasc)	Cardiovascular/calcium antagonist
amoxicillin trihydrate (Amoxil, Trimox)	Antibiotic/penicillin
amoxicillin+ clavulanate (Augmentin)	Antibiotic/penicillin
anastrozole (Arimidex)	Endocrine/aromatase inhibitor

Chart continued on following page

---

*From Chabner D-E: The Language of Medicine, 7th ed. Philadelphia, WB Saunders, 2004.

177

Generic (Brand Name)	Explanation of Use
aspirin	Analgesic/mild; antiplatelet
atenolol (Tenormin)	Cardiovascular/beta-blocker
atorvastatin (Lipitor)	Cardiovascular/cholesterol-lowering
azithromycin (Zithromax)	Antibiotic/erythromycin class
beclomethasone (Vanceril)	Respiratory/steroid inhaler
buspirone (BuSpar)	Tranquilizer/minor
butabarbital (Butisol)	Sedative/hypnotic
caffeine	Stimulant
carbamazepine (Tegretol)	Anticonvulsant
cefprozil (Cefzil)	Antibiotic/cephalosporin
ceftazidine (Fortaz)	Antibiotic/cephalosporin
cefuroxime axetil (Ceftin)	Antibiotic/cephalosporin
celecoxib (Celebrex)	Analgesic/NSAID
cephalexin (Keflex)	Antibiotic/cephalosporin
cetirizine (Zyrtec)	Antihistamine
chlorpheniramine maleate (Chlor-Trimeton)	Antihistamine
chlorpromazine (Thorazine)	Tranquilizer/major/phenothiazine
cholestyramine (Questran)	Cardiovascular/cholesterol-lowering
cimetidine (Tagamet)	GI/antiulcer/anti-GERD
ciprofloxacin (Cipro)	Antibiotic/quinolone
cisapride (Propulsid)	GI/antiulcer/anti-GERD
clarithromycin (Biaxin)	Antibiotic/erythromycin class
codeine	Analgesic/narcotic
dextroamphetamine sulfate (Dexedrine)	Stimulant
diazepam (Valium)	Tranquilizer/minor/benzodiazepine
diclofenac (Voltaren)	Analgesic/NSAID

Generic (Brand Name)	Explanation of Use
digoxin (Lanoxin)	Cardiovascular/anti-CHF
diltiazem (Cardizem CD)	Cardiovascular/calcium antagonist
diphenhydramine (Benadryl)	Antihistamine
diphenoxylate+ atropine (Lomotil)	GI/antidiarrheal
doxycycline	Antibiotic/tetracycline
enalapril maleate (Vasotec)	Cardiovascular ACE inhibitor
enoxaparin sodium (Lovenox)	Anticoagulant
epinephrine	Bronchodilator
erythromycin (Ery-Tab)	Antibiotic/erythromycin
estrogen (Premarin, Prempro, Estradiol)	Endocrine/estrogen
ether	Anesthetic/general
extended insulin zinc suspension (Ultralente)	Antidiabetic/type 1
famotidine (Pepcid)	GI/antiulcer/anti-GERD
felbamate (Felbatol)	Anticonvulsant
fexofenadine (Allegra)	Antihistamine
flecainide (Tambocor)	Cardiovascular/ antiarrhythmic
fluconazole (Diflucan)	Antifungal
flunisolide (AeroBid)	Respiratory/steroid inhaler
fluoxymesterone (Halotestin)	Endocrine/androgen
flutamide (Eulexin)	Endocrine/antiandrogen
fluticasone propionate (Flovent)	Respiratory/steroid inhaler
fluvastatin (Lescol)	Cardiovascular/cholesterol-lowering
fulvestrant (Faslodex)	Endocrine/aromatase inhibitor

Chart continued on following page

Generic (Brand Name)	Explanation of Use
furosemide (Lasix)	Cardiovascular/diuretic
gabapentin (Neurontin)	Anticonvulsant
glipizide (Glucotrol XL)	Antidiabetic/type 2/ sulfonylurea
glyburide	Antidiabetic/type 2/ sulfonylurea
halothane (Fluothane)	Anesthetic/general
human insulin (Humalog)	Antidiabetic/type 1
human insulin NPH (Humulin N)	Antidiabetic/type 1
hydrochlorothiazide (Diuril)	Cardiovascular/diuretic
hydrocodone w/APAP	Analgesic/narcotic
hydromorphone (Dilaudid)	Analgesic/narcotic
ibuprofen (Motrin, Advil)	Analgesic/NSAID
indinavir (Crixivan)	Antiviral/protease inhibitor/anti-HIV
insulin zinc suspension (Lente)	Antidiabetic/type 1
interferon (Alfa-n1) (Wellferon)	Antiviral/anti-cancer drug
ipratropium bromide + albuterol (Atrovent)	Bronchodilator
irbesartan (Avapro)	Cardiovascular/angiotensin II receptor antagonist
isoniazid or INH (Nydrazid)	Antitubercular
lamivudine (Epivir)	Antiviral/reverse transcriptase inhibitor/anti-HIV
lansoprazole (Prevacid)	GI/antiulcer/anti-GERD
letrozole (Femara)	Endocrine/aromatase inhibitor
levothyroxine (Levoxyl, Levothroid, Synthroid)	Endocrine/thyroid hormone

Generic (Brand Name)	Explanation of Use
lidocaine (Xylocaine)	Anesthetic/local
lidocaine+prilocaine (EMLA)	Anesthetic/local
liothyronine (Cytomel)	Endocrine/thyroid hormone
liotrix (Thyrolar)	Endocrine/thyroid hormone
lisinopril (Prinivil, Zestril)	Cardiovascular/ACE inhibitor
lithium carbonate (Eskalith)	Tranquilizer/major
loperamide (Imodium)	GI/antidiarrheal
loratadine (Claritin)	Antihistamine
lorazepam (Ativan)	Tranquilizer/minor/ benzodiazepine
losartan potassium (Cozaar)	Cardiovascular/angiotensin II receptor antagonist
lovastatin (Mevacor)	Cardiovascular/cholesterol- lowering
magnesium antacid (milk of magnesia)	GI/antacid
meclizine (Antivert)	Antihistamine
medroxyprogesterone acetate (Cycrin, Provera)	Endocrine/progestin
megestrol (Megace)	Endocrine/progestin
meperidine (Demerol)	Analgesic/narcotic
metaproterenol (Alupent)	Bronchodilator
metformin (Glucophage)	Antidiabetic/type 2/biguanide
methylphenidate (Ritalin)	Stimulant
methylprednisolone (Medrol)	Respiratory/steroid IV or oral
methyltestosterone (Virilon)	Endocrine/androgen
metoclopramide (Reglan)	GI/antinauseant

Chart continued on following page

Generic (Brand Name)	Explanation of Use
metoprolol (Lopressor, Toprol-XL)	Cardiovascular/beta-blocker
miconazole (Monistat)	Antifungal
modafinil (Provigil)	Stimulant/sleep antagonist
montelukast (Singulair)	Respiratory/leukotriene modifier
nafcillin (Unipen)	Antibiotic/penicillin
naproxen (Naprosyn, Aleve)	Analgesic/NSAID
nifedipine (Adalat CC, Procardia)	Cardiovascular/calcium antagonist
nilutamide (Casodex)	Endocrine/antiandrogen
nitrofurantoin (Macrobid)	Antibiotic/sulfonamide
nitroglycerin	Cardiovascular/antianginal
nitrous oxide	Anesthetic/general
nystatin (Nilstat)	Antifungal
ofloxacin (Floxin)	Antibiotic/quinolone
olanzapine (Zyprexa)	Tranquilizer/major/antipsychotic
omeprazole (Prilosec)	GI/antiulcer/anti-GERD
ondansetron (Zofran)	GI/antinauseant
oxacillin (Bactocill)	Antibiotic/penicillin
oxycodone (Oxycontin)	Analgesic/narcotic
pamidronate disodium (Aredia)	Anti-osteoporosis/bisphosphonate
paregoric	GI/antidiarrheal
phenergan (Promethazine)	GI/antinauseant; antihistamine
phenobarbital	Sedative/hypnotic; anticonvulsant
phenytoin sodium (Dilantin)	Anticonvulsant
pioglitazone (Actos)	Antidiabetic/type 2
pravastatin (Pravachol)	Cardiovascular/cholesterol-lowering
prednisone	Respiratory/steroid IV or oral
protamine zinc suspension (PZI)	Antidiabetic/type 1

Generic (Brand Name)	Explanation of Use
procainamide (Pronestyl)	Cardiovascular/antiarrhythmic
procaine (Novocaine)	Anesthetic/local
prochlorperazine maleate (Compazine)	GI/antinauseant
propoxyphene (Darvon)	Analgesic/narcotic
propranolol (Inderal)	Cardiovascular/beta-blocker
quinapril (Accupril)	Cardiovascular/ACE inhibitor
raloxifene HCl (Evista)	Endocrine/antiosteoporosis
ramipril (Altace)	Cardiovascular/ACE inhibitor
ranitidine (Zantac)	GI/antiulcer/anti-GERD
repaglinide (Prandin)	Antidiabetic/type 2/ meglitinide
rifampin (Rifadin)	Antitubercular
rofecoxib (Vioxx)	Analgesic/NSAID
rosiglitazone (Avandia)	Antidiabetic/type 2
salmeterol (Serevent)	Bronchodilator
simvastatin (Zocor)	Cardiovascular/cholesterol-lowering
sotalol (Betapace)	Cardiovascular/beta-blocker
spironolactone (Aldactone)	Cardiovascular/diuretic
sulfamethoxazole+ trimethoprim (Bactrim)	Antibiotic/sulfonamide
sulfisoxazole (Gantrisin)	Antibiotic/sulfonamide
tamoxifen (Nolvadex)	Endocrine/antiestrogen
temazepam (Restoril)	Sedative/hypnotic/ benzodiazepine
terbinafine (Lamisil)	Antifungal
tetracycline	Antibiotic/tetracycline
theophylline (Theo-Dur)	Bronchodilator
thiopental (Pentothal)	Anesthetic/general
thioridazine (Mellaril)	Tranquilizer/major/ phenothiazine

Chart continued on following page

Generic (Brand Name)	Explanation of Use
tissue plasminogen activator (tPA)	Anticoagulant
tramadol (Ultram)	Analgesic/mild
triamcinolone (Azmacort)	Respiratory/steroid inhaler
triamterene (Dyazide)	Cardiovascular/diuretic
triazolam (Halcion)	Sedative/hypnotic/benzodiazepine
trifluoperazine (Stelazine)	Tranquilizer/major/phenothiazine
valproic acid (Depakote)	Anticonvulsant
warfarin (Coumadin)	Anticoagulant
zafirlukast (Accolate)	Respiratory/leukotriene modifier
zidovudine or AZT (Retrovir)	Antiviral/reverse transcriptase inhibitor/anti-HIV
zileuton (Zyflo Filmtab)	Respiratory/leukotriene modifier
zoledronic acid (Zometa)	Antiosteoporosis/bisphosphonate
zolpidem tartrate (Ambien)	Sedative/hypnotic

The Top 100 Prescription Drugs (Listed Alphabetically)*[1]

Trade Name[2]	Generic Name	Type/Use	Rank[3]
Accupril	quinapril	Antihypertensive (ACE inhibitor)	55
Actos	pioglitazone	Antidiabetic agent	96
Advair Diskus	fluticasone/salmeterol	Bronchodilator	73
Allegra	fexofenadine	Antihistamine	24
Altace	ramipril	Antihypertensive (ACE inhibitor)	77

* Adapted from Mosby's Drug Consult, 2002, **www.mosbysdrugconsult.com.**
[1] Based on data from Scott-Levin, Newton, Pa.
[2] Names in parentheses in this column are the most recognizable trade names for drugs that are available generically.
[3] Names in parentheses in this column are the different manufacturers of the same drug, each next to their respective ranking within the top 100.

Chart continued on following page

The Top 100 Prescription Drugs (Listed Alphabetically) Continued

Trade Name[2]	Generic Name	Type/Use	Rank[3]
Ambien	zolpidem	Sedative-hypnotic (for insomnia)	32
Amoxil	amoxicillin	Antibiotic (penicillin-type)	70 5
Ativan	lorazepam	Anxiolytic; benzodiazepine	35
Augmentin	amoxicillin/clavulanate	Antibiotic (penicillin-type)	43
Avandia	rosiglitazone	Antidiabetic agent	95
Bactrim	sulfamethoxazole/trimethoprim	Antibiotic	53
Bancap-HC	acetaminophen	Analgesic	1
Calan	verapamil SR	Antiarrhythmic; calcium channel blocker	72

The Top 100 Prescription Drugs (Listed Alphabetically) *Continued*

Trade Name[2]	Generic Name	Type/Use	Rank[3]
Catapres-TTS	clonidine	Antiadrenergic	91
Celebrex	celecoxib	Analgesic	20
Celexa	citalopram	Antidepressant	28
Cipro	ciprofloxacin	Anti-infective (quinolone-type)	56
Clarinex	desloratadine	Antihistamine	87
Claritin	loratadine	Antihistamine and decongestant	38
Coumadin tablets	warfarin tablets	Anticoagulant	82 64

Chart continued on following page

The Top 100 Prescription Drugs (Listed Alphabetically) *Continued*

Trade Name[2]	Generic Name	Type/Use	Rank[3]
Cozaar	losartan	Antihypertensive (Angiotension II receptor antagonist)	92
Deltasone	prednisone oral	Corticosteroid	25
Desyrel	trazodone	Antidepressant	57
Diflucan	fluconazole	Antifungal	67
Diovan	valsartan	Angiotensin II receptor antagonist	78
Dyazide	HCTZ/triamterene	Diuretic	21
Effexor XR	venlafaxine extended release	Antidepressant	48
Elavil	amitriptyline	Antidepressant	42

The Top 100 Prescription Drugs (Listed Alphabetically) *Continued*

Trade Name[2]	Generic Name	Type/Use	Rank[3]
Esidrix	hydrochlorothiazide	Diuretic	11
Estraderm	estradiol oral	Hormone (estrogen)	94
Flexeril	cyclobenzaprine	Musculoskeletal relaxant	61
Flonase	fluticasone	Corticosteroid	60
Flovent	fluticasone	Corticosteroid	100
Fosamax	alendronate	Bone resorption inhibitor; calcium inhibitor	36
Glucophage	metformin	Antidiabetic (biguanide antihyperglycemic)	37

Chart continued on following page

The Top 100 Prescription Drugs (Listed Alphabetically) *Continued*

Trade Name[2]	Generic Name	Type/Use	Rank[3]
Glucotrol XL	glipizide	Oral sulfonylurea (antidiabetic)	68
Ismo	isosorbide mononitrate	Vasodilator	80
Keflex	cephalexin	Antibiotic	16
Klonopin	clonazepam	Anxiolytic/benzodiazepine	54
Lanoxin	digoxin	Cardiotonic and antiarrhythmic	84
Lasix	furosemide oral	Diuretic	7
Levaquin	levofloxacin	Antibiotic	65
Levoxyl	levothyroxine	Thyroid hormone	22
Lipitor	atorvastatin	Cholesterol lowering agent	2

The Top 100 Prescription Drugs (Listed Alphabetically) *Continued*

Trade Name[2]	Generic Name	Type/Use	Rank[3]
Lopressor	metoprolol tartrate	Antiadrenergic	34
Lotensin	benazepril	Antihypertensive (ACE inhibitor)	89
Lotrel	amlodipine/benazepril	Angiotensin converting enzyme inhibitors	79
Medrol	methylprednisolone tablets	Corticosteroid	86
Micronase	glyburide	Antidiabetic agent	75
Motrin	ibuprofen	Analgesic (non-narcotic)	19
Naprosyn	naproxen	Nonsteroidal anti-inflammatory drug (NSAID)	58

Chart continued on following page

191

The Top 100 Prescription Drugs (Listed Alphabetically) *Continued*

Trade Name[2]	Generic Name	Type/Use	Rank[3]
Nasonex	mometasone	Corticosteroid	90
Neurontin	gabapentin	Anticonvulsant	45
Nexium	esomeprazole	Gastrointestinal	52
Norvasc	amlodipine	Antihypertensive (calcium channel blocker)	8
Ortho Tri-Cyclen	low-dose estrogen/ low-dose progestin	Pregnancy prevention (contraceptive)	23
Paxil	paroxetine	Antidepressant	13
Percocet	APAP oxycodone	Analgesic	83
Plavix	clopidogrel	Platelet inhibitor	69

The Top 100 Prescription Drugs (Listed Alphabetically) *Continued*

Trade Name[2]	Generic Name	Type/Use	Rank[3]
Pravachol	pravastatin	Cholesterol lowering agent	50
Premarin	estrogen	Hormone (female)	6
Prempro	conjugated estrogen/ medroxyprogesterone	Hormone (female) (HRT)	46
Prevacid	lansoprazole	Gastric acid pump inhibitor	18
Prilosec	omeprazole	Gastric acid pump inhibitor	29
Prinivil	lisinopril	Antihypertensive (ACE inhibitor)	97
Protonix	pantoprazole	Protein pump inhibitor	71
Prozac	fluoxetine	Antidepressant (SSRI)	30

Chart continued on following page

The Top 100 Prescription Drugs (Listed Alphabetically) *Continued*

Trade Name[2]	Generic Name	Type/Use	Rank[3]
Risperdal	risperidone	Antipsychotic	74
Singulair	montelukast	Leukotriene	51
Slow-K	potassium chloride	Electrolyte	59 62
Soma	carisoprodol	Musculoskeletal relaxant	74
Synthroid	levothyroxine	Thyroid hormone	3
Tenormin	atenolol	Antiadrenergic; beta-blocker	4
Toprol-XL	metoprolol	Antihypertensive (beta-blocker)	26
Trimox	amoxicillin	Antibiotic (penicillin-type)	39

The Top 100 Prescription Drugs (Listed Alphabetically) *Continued*

Trade Name[2]	Generic Name	Type/Use	Rank[3]
Tylenol w/ codeine	APAP codeine	Analgesic	27
Valium	diazepam	Anxiolytic/benzodiazepine	66
Vasotec	enalapril	Antihypertensive (ACE inhibitor)	63
Veetids	penicillin VK	Antibiotic (penicillin-type)	93
Ventolin	albuterol	Bronchodilator	9 85
Vexol	rimexolone	Corticosteroid	99
Viagra	sildenafil citrate	Vasodilator (for erectile dysfunction)	40

Chart continued on following page

The Top 100 Prescription Drugs (Listed Alphabetically) *Continued*

Trade Name[2]	Generic Name	Type/Use	Rank[3]
Vibramycin	doxycycline	Antibiotic	76
Vioxx	rofecoxib	Analgesic (nonnarcotic) for arthritis	31
Wellbutrin SR	bupropion	Antidepressant; smoking cessation aid	44
Wygesic	APAP/propoxyphene-N	Analgesic	14
Xanax	alprazolam	Anxiolytic/benzodiazepine	10
Zantac	ranitidine	Antihistamine/gastrointestinal	41
Zestril	lisinopril	Antihypertensive (ACE inhibitor)	47 49
Zithromax Susp	azithromycin	Antibiotic (erythromycin-type)	81

The Top 100 Prescription Drugs (Listed Alphabetically) *Continued*

Trade Name[2]	Generic Name	Type/Use	Rank[3]
Zithromax Z-Pack	azithromycin	Antibiotic (erythromycin-type)	15
Zocor	simvastatin	Cholesterol lowering agent	17
Zoloft	sertraline	Antidepressant (SSRI)	12
Zyloprim	allopurinol	Antigout agent	88
Zyrtec	cetirizine	Antihistamine	33

ACE = angiotensin-converting enzyme
APAP = acetaminophen
BPH = benign prostatic hyperplasia

CHF = congestive heart failure
GERD = gastroesophageal reflux disease
HCTZ = hydrochlorothiazide

N = napsylate
NPH = isophane insulin
SSRI = selective serotonin receptor inhibitor

The Top 100 Principal Diagnoses and Associated Principal Procedures*

Diagnosis	Most Common Associated Principal Procedures
1. Liveborn	• Circumcision • Prophylactic vaccinations and inoculations • Respiratory intubation and mechanical ventilation
2. Coronary atherosclerosis and other heart disease	• Percutaneous transluminal coronary angioplasty • Coronary artery bypass graft • Diagnostic cardiac catheterization, coronary arteriography • Cardiac stress tests
3. Pneumonia (except that caused by tuberculosis or sexually transmitted diseases)	• Diagnostic bronchoscopy and biopsy of bronchus • Respiratory intubation and mechanical ventilation

*Source: Agency for Health Care Policy and Research, Center for Organization and Delivery Studies, Healthcare Cost and Utilization Project (HCUP).

Chart continued on following page

The Top 100 Principal Diagnoses and Associated Principal Procedures *Continued*

Diagnosis	Most Common Associated Procedures
4. Congestive heart failure, nonhypertensive	• Diagnostic cardiac catheterization, coronary arteriography • Diagnostic ultrasound of heart (echocardiogram) • Respiratory intubation and mechanical ventilation • Incision of pleura, thoracentesis, chest drainage
5. Acute myocardial infarction	• Percutaneous transluminal coronary angioplasty • Diagnostic cardiac catheterization, coronary arteriography • Coronary artery bypass graft
6. Trauma to perineum and vulva	• Repair of current obstetrical laceration • Episiotomy • Forceps, vacuum, and breech delivery • Ligation of fallopian tubes
7. Acute cerebrovascular disease	• CT scan (head) • Respiratory intubation and mechanical ventilation • Gastrostomy, temporary and permanent • Magnetic resonance imaging

The Top 100 Principal Diagnoses and Associated Principal Procedures *Continued*

Diagnosis	Most Common Associated Procedures
8. Normal pregnancy and/or delivery	• Episiotomy • Artificial rupture of membranes to assist delivery • Ligation of fallopian tubes
9. Affective disorders	• Psychological and psychiatric evaluation and therapy • Alcohol and drug rehabilitation/detoxification • CT scan (head)
10. Cardiac dysrhythmias	• Insertion, revision, replacement, removal of cardiac pacemaker or cardioverter/defibrillator • Conversion of cardiac rhythm • Diagnostic ultrasound of heart (echocardiogram)
11. Chronic obstructive pulmonary disease and bronchiectasis	• Respiratory intubation and mechanical ventilation • Diagnostic bronchoscopy and biopsy of bronchus • Arterial blood gases

Chart continued on following page

The Top 100 Principal Diagnoses and Associated Principal Procedures *Continued*

Diagnosis	Most Common Associated Procedures
12. Spondylosis, intervertebral disk disorders, other back problems	• Laminectomy, excision intervertebral disk • Spinal fusion • Insertion of catheter or spinal stimulator and injection into spinal canal • Myelogram
13. Nonspecific chest pain	• Diagnostic cardiac catheterization, coronary arteriography • Cardiac stress tests • Diagnostic ultrasound of heart (echocardiogram) • Electrographic cardiac monitoring
14. Fluid and electrolyte disorders	• Upper gastrointestinal endoscopy, biopsy • Gastrostomy, temporary and permanent • CT scan (head)
15. Biliary tract disease	• Cholecystectomy and common duct exploration • Endoscopic retrograde cannulation of pancreas (ERCP)

The Top 100 Principal Diagnoses and Associated Principal Procedures *Continued*

Diagnosis	Most Common Associated Procedures
16. Complication of device, implant or graft	• Hip replacement, total and partial • Creation, revision, and removal of arteriovenous fistula or vessel-to-vessel cannula for dialysis • Percutaneous transluminal coronary angioplasty (PTCA)
17. Fetal distress and abnormal forces of labor	• Cesarean section • Forceps, vacuum, and breech delivery • Episiotomy • Repair of current obstetrical laceration
18. Septicemia (except in labor)	• Diagnostic spinal tap • Blood transfusion • Debridement of wound, infection or burn
19. Asthma	• Respiratory intubation and mechanical ventilation • Arterial blood gases
20. Osteoarthritis	• Arthroplasty knee • Hip replacement, total and partial • Arthroplasty other than hip or knee

Chart continued on following page

Diagnosis	Most Common Associated Procedures
21. Urinary tract infections	• Endoscopy and endoscopic biopsy of the urinary tract • Diagnostic ultrasound of urinary tract • Diagnostic spinal tap
22. Diabetes mellitus with complications	• Amputation of lower extremity • Debridement of wound, infection, or burn • Peripheral vascular bypass
23. Other complications of birth, puerperium affecting management of mother	• Episiotomy • Repair of current obstetrical laceration • Forceps, vacuum, and breech delivery • Cesarean section
24. Fracture of neck of femur	• Treatment, fracture or dislocation of hip and femur • Hip replacement, total and partial • Physical therapy exercises, manipulation, and other procedures
25. Other complications of pregnancy	• Traction, splints, and other wound care • Episiotomy • Cesarean section • Repair of current obstetrical laceration

The Top 100 Principal Diagnoses and Associated Principal Procedures *Continued*

Diagnosis	Most Common Associated Procedures
26. Rehabilitation care, fitting of prostheses, and adjustment of devices	• Physical therapy exercises, manipulation, and other procedures • Diagnostic physical therapy
27. Complications of surgical procedures or medical care	• Debridement of wound, infection, or burn • Incision and drainage, skin and subcutaneous tissue • Incision of pleura, thoracentesis, chest drainage
28. Skin and subcutaneous tissue infections	• Incision and drainage, skin and subcutaneous tissue • Debridement of wound, infection, or burn
29. Gastrointestinal hemorrhage	• Upper gastrointestinal endoscopy, biopsy • Colonoscopy and biopsy • Blood transfusion
30. Alcohol-related mental disorders	• Alcohol and drug rehabilitation/detoxification • Psychological and psychiatric evaluation and therapy • CT scan (head) • Respiratory intubation and mechanical ventilation

Chart continued on following page

The Top 100 Principal Diagnoses and Associated Principal Procedures *Continued*

Diagnosis	Most Common Associated Procedures
31. Intestinal obstruction without hernia	• Excision, lysis peritoneal adhesions • Small bowel resection • Colonoscopy and biopsy • Nasogastric tube
32. Fracture of lower limb	• Treatment, fracture or dislocation of lower extremity (other than hip or femur) • Treatment, fracture or dislocation of hip and femur • Traction, splints, and other wound care • Debridement of wound, infection, or burn
33. Early or threatened labor	• Cesarean section • Episiotomy • Fetal monitoring
34. Previous cesarean section	• Cesarean section • Episiotomy • Forceps, vacuum, and breech delivery • Repair of current obstetrical laceration

The Top 100 Principal Diagnoses and Associated Principal Procedures *Continued*

Diagnosis	Most Common Associated Procedures
35. Umbilical cord complication	• Episiotomy • Repair of current obstetrical laceration • Forceps, vacuum, and breech delivery • Artificial rupture of membranes to assist delivery
36. Secondary malignancies	• Incision of pleura, thoracentesis, chest drainage • Therapeutic radiology • Cancer chemotherapy
37. Maintenance chemotherapy, radiotherapy	• Cancer chemotherapy • Therapeutic radiology
38. Schizophrenia and related disorders	• Psychological and psychiatric evaluation and therapy • Alcohol and drug rehabilitation/detoxification • CT scan (head)

Chart continued on following page

The Top 100 Principal Diagnoses and Associated Principal Procedures *Continued*

Diagnosis	Most Common Associated Procedures
39. Hypertension with complications and secondary hypertension	• Hemodialysis • Creation, revision and removal of arteriovenous fistula or vessel-to-vessel cannula for dialysis • Diagnostic cardiac catheterization, coronary arteriography • Diagnostic ultrasound of heart (echocardiogram)
40. Substance-related mental disorders	• Alcohol and drug rehabilitation/detoxification • Psychological and psychiatric evaluation and therapy • CT scan (head) • Diagnostic spinal tap
41. Diverticulosis and diverticulitis	• Colorectal resection • Colonoscopy and biopsy • Upper gastrointestinal endoscopy, biopsy • CT scan (abdomen)
42. Benign neoplasm of uterus	• Hysterectomy, abdominal and vaginal • Diagnostic dilatation and curettage • Oophorectomy, unilateral and bilateral

The Top 100 Principal Diagnoses and Associated Principal Procedures *Continued*

Diagnosis	Most Common Associated Procedures
43. Appendicitis and other appendiceal conditions	• Appendectomy • Colorectal resection • Excision, lysis peritoneal adhesions
44. Epilepsy, convulsions	• CT scan (head) • Respiratory intubation and mechanical ventilation • Diagnostic spinal tap • Electroencephalogram (EEG)
45. Polyhydramnios and other problems of amniotic caviy	• Episiotomy • Cesarean section • Repair of current obstetrical laceration • Forceps, vacuum, and breech delivery
46. Acute bronchitis	• Diagnostic spinal tap • Diagnostic bronchoscopy and biopsy of bronchus

Chart continued on following page

The Top 100 Principal Diagnoses and Associated Principal Procedures *Continued*

Diagnosis	Most Common Associated Procedures
47. Respiratory failure, insufficiency, arrest	• Respiratory intubation and mechanical ventilation • Tracheostomy, temporary and permanent • Diagnostic bronchoscopy and biopsy of bronchus
48. Pancreatic disorders (not diabetes)	• Cholecystectomy and common duct exploration • Upper gastrointestinal endoscopy, biopsy • Endoscopic retrograde cannulation of pancreas (ERCP)
49. Transient cerebral ischemia	• CT scan (head) • Diagnostic ultrasound of heart (echocardiogram) • Diagnostic ultrasound of head and neck • Magnetic resonance imaging
50. Syncope	• CT scan (head) • Diagnostic ultrasound of heart (echocardiogram)
51. Phlebitis, thrombophlebitis and thromboembolism	• Arteriogram or venogram (not heart and head)

The Top 100 Principal Diagnoses and Associated Principal Procedures *Continued*

Diagnosis	Most Common Associated Procedures
52. Calculus of urinary tract	• Transurethral excision, drainage, or removal of urinary obstruction • Ureteral catheterization • Intravenous pyelogram • Endoscopy and endoscopic biopsy of the urinary tract
53. Hypertension complicating pregnancy, childbirth and the puerperium	• Cesarean section • Episiotomy • Forceps, vacuum, and breech delivery
54. Aspiration pneumonitis, food/vomitus	• Respiratory intubation and mechanical ventilation • Gastrostomy, temporary and permanent • Upper gastrointestinal endoscopy, biopsy • Diagnostic bronchoscopy and biopsy of bronchus
55. Occlusion or stenosis of precerebral arteries	• Endarterectomy, vessel of head and neck • Cerebral arteriogram • CT scan (head)

Chart continued on following page

The Top 100 Principal Diagnoses and Associated Principal Procedures *Continued*

Diagnosis	Most Common Associated Procedures
56. Intracranial injury	• CT scan (head) • Suture of skin and subcutaneous tissue • Incision and excision of central nervous system (CNS) • Respiratory intubation and mechanical ventilation
57. Other fractures	• Suture of skin and subcutaneous tissue • Physical therapy exercises, manipulation, and other procedures
58. Other lower respiratory disease	• Diagnostic bronchoscopy and biopsy of bronchus • Diagnostic cardiac catheterization, coronary arteriography • Lobectomy or pneumonectomy
59. Abdominal hernia	• Inguinal and femoral hernia repair • Excision, lysis peritoneal adhesions
60. Cancer of bronchus, lung	• Lobectomy or pneumonectomy • Diagnostic bronchoscopy and biopsy of bronchus • Incision of pleura, thoracentesis, chest drainage • Therapeutic radiology

The Top 100 Principal Diagnoses and Associated Principal Procedures *Continued*

Diagnosis	Most Common Associated Procedures
61. Esophageal disorders	• Upper gastrointestinal endoscopy, biopsy • Diagnostic cardiac catheterization, coronary arteriography • Esophageal dilatation
62. Prolapse of female genital organs	• Hysterectomy, abdominal and vaginal • Repair of cystocele and rectocele, obliteration of vaginal vault • Genitourinary incontinence procedures • Oophorectomy, unilateral and bilateral
63. Malposition, malpresentation	• Cesarean section • Forceps, vacuum, and breech delivery • Episiotomy • Repair of current obstetrical laceration
64. Other gastrointestinal disorders	• Colonoscopy and biopsy • Colorectal resection • Upper gastrointestinal endoscopy, biopsy

Chart continued on following page

The Top 100 Principal Diagnoses and Associated Principal Procedures *Continued*

Diagnosis	Most Common Associated Procedures
65. Abdominal pain	• Upper gastrointestinal endoscopy, biopsy • Appendectomy • CT scan (abdomen) • Colonoscopy and biopsy
66. Other and unspecified benign neoplasm	• Oophorectomy, unilateral and bilateral • Hysterectomy, abdominal and vaginal • Thyroidectomy, partial or complete • Colorectal resection
67. Fetopelvic disproportion, obstruction	• Cesarean section • Forceps, vacuum, and breech delivery • Episiotomy • Repair of current obstetrical laceration
68. Other mental conditions	• Psychological and psychiatric evaluation and therapy • Alcohol and drug rehabilitation/detoxification • Suture of skin and subcutaneous tissue

The Top 100 Principal Diagnoses and Associated Principal Procedures *Continued*

Diagnosis	Most Common Associated Procedures
69. Gastritis and duodenitis	• Upper gastrointestinal endoscopy, biopsy • Colonoscopy and biopsy • Blood transfusion
70. Fracture of upper limb	• Treatment, fracture or dislocation of radius and ulna • Arthroplasty other than hip or knee • Traction, splints, and other wound care
71. Peripheral and visceral atherosclerosis	• Peripheral vascular bypass • Colonoscopy and biopsy • Colorectal resection
72. Senility and organic mental disorders	• CT scan (head) • Psychological and psychiatric evaluation and therapy • Diagnostic spinal tap • Magnetic resonance imaging
73. Noninfectious gastroenteritis	• Colonoscopy and biopsy • Upper gastrointestinal endoscopy, biopsy • CT scan (abdomen)

Chart continued on following page

The Top 100 Principal Diagnoses and Associated Principal Procedures *Continued*

Diagnosis	Most Common Associated Procedures
74. HIV infection	• Diagnostic bronchoscopy and biopsy of bronchus • Diagnostic spinal tap • Blood transfusion
75. Cancer of breast	• Mastectomy • Lumpectomy, quadrantectomy of breast • Breast biopsy and other diagnostic procedures on breast
76. Poisoning by other medications and drugs	• Respiratory intubation and mechanical ventilation • Electrographic cardiac monitoring • CT scan (head)
77. Intestinal infection	• Colonoscopy and biopsy • Upper gastrointestinal endoscopy, biopsy • Diagnostic spinal tap
78. Hyperplasia of prostate	• Transurethral resection of prostate • Open prostatectomy • Endoscopy and endoscopic biopsy of the urinary tract • Procedures on the urethra

The Top 100 Principal Diagnoses and Associated Principal Procedures *Continued*

Diagnosis	Most Common Associated Procedures
79. Cancer of colon	• Colorectal resection • Colonoscopy and biopsy • Upper gastrointestinal endoscopy, biopsy
80. Other female genital disorders	• Hysterectomy, abdominal and vaginal • Genitourinary incontinence procedures • Oophorectomy, unilateral and bilateral
81. Cancer of prostate	• Open prostatectomy • Transurethral resection of prostate
82. Other nervous system disorders	• Diagnostic spinal tap • CT scan (head) • Magnetic resonance imaging
83. Forceps delivery	• Forceps, vacuum, and breech delivery • Repair of current obstetrical laceration • Episiotomy

Chart continued on following page

The Top 100 Principal Diagnoses and Associated Principal Procedures *Continued*

Diagnosis	Most Common Associated Procedures
84. Other connective tissue disease	• Arthroplasty other than hip or knee • Debridement of wound, infection or burn
85. Pleurisy, pneumothorax, pulmonary collapse	• Incision of pleura, thoracentesis, chest drainage • Lobectomy or pneumonectomy • Diagnostic bronchoscopy and biopsy of bronchus
86. Viral infection	• Diagnostic spinal tap • Upper gastrointestinal endoscopy, biopsy • CT scan (head)
87. Prolonged pregnancy	• Episiotomy • Cesarean section • Forceps, vacuum, and breech delivery • Repair of current obstetrical laceration
88. Deficiency and other anemia	• Blood transfusion • Upper gastrointestinal endoscopy, biopsy • Bone marrow biopsy • Colonoscopy and biopsy

The Top 100 Principal Diagnoses and Associated Principal Procedures *Continued*

Diagnosis	Most Common Associated Procedures
89. Crushing injury or internal injury	• Incision of pleura, thoracentesis, chest drainage
90. Heart valve disorders	• Heart valve procedures • Diagnostic cardiac catheterization, coronary arteriography • Diagnostic ultrasound of heart (echocardiogram)
91. Other circulatory disease	• Peripheral vascular bypass • Diagnostic cardiac catheterization, coronary arteriography
92. Acute and unspecified renal failure	• Hemodialysis • Creation, revision and removal of arteriovenous fistula or vessel-to-vessel cannula for dialysis • Upper gastrointestinal endoscopy, biopsy
93. Endometriosis	• Hysterectomy, abdominal and vaginal • Oophorectomy, unilateral and bilateral
94. Other bone disease and musculoskeletal deformities	• Hip replacement, total and partial • Spinal fusion • Partial excision bone

Chart continued on following page

The Top 100 Principal Diagnoses and Associated Principal Procedures *Continued*

Diagnosis	Most Common Associated Procedures
95. Sprains and strains	• Arthroplasty knee • Arthroplasty other than hip or knee
96. Other upper respiratory infections	• Diagnostic spinal tap
97. Pulmonary heart disease	• Radioisotope pulmonary scan • Arteriogram or venogram (not heart and head) • Diagnostic cardiac catheterization, coronary arteriography
98. Pericarditis, endocarditis, and myocarditis, cardiomyopathy (except that caused by tuberculosis or sexually transmitted diseases)	• Diagnostic cardiac catheterization, coronary arteriography • Diagnostic ultrasound of heart (echocardiogram)
99. Aortic, peripheral, and visceral artery aneurysms	• Aortic resection, replacement or anastomosis • Peripheral vascular bypass
100. Other injuries and conditions due to external causes	• Upper gastrointestinal endoscopy, biopsy • CT scan (head) • Nonoperative removal of foreign body • Respiratory intubation and mechanical ventilation

Normal Hematological Reference Values and Implications of Abnormal Results*

The implications of abnormal results are major ones in each category. SI units are the International System of Units that are generally accepted for all scientific and technical uses.

cu mm = cubic millimeter (mm^3)

dL = deciliter (1/10 liter or 100 mL)

g = gram

L = liter

mg = milligram (1/1000 gram)

mL = milliliter

mEq = milliequivalent

mill = million

mm = millimeter (1/1000 meter)

mmol = millimole

thou = thousand

U = unit

μl = microliter

μmol = micromole (one-millionth of a mole)

*From Chabner D-E: The Language of Medicine, 7th ed. Philadelphia, WB Saunders, 2004.

Cell Counts*

	Conventional Units	SI Units	Implications
Erythrocytes (RBC)			*High* • Polycythemia
Females	4.0–5.5 million/mm³ or μl	4.0–5.5×10^{12}/L	• Dehydration
Males	4.5–6.0 million/mm³ or μl	4.5–6.0×10^{12}/L	*Low* • Iron deficiency anemia
			• Blood loss
Leukocytes (WBC)			*High* • Bacterial infection
Total	5000–10,000/mm³ or μl	5.0–10.0×10^9/L	• Leukemia
			• Eosinophils high in allergy

Chart continued on following page

*From Chabner D-E: The Language of Medicine, 7th ed. Philadelphia, WB Saunders, 2004.

Cell Counts *Continued*

	Conventional Units	SI Units	Implications	
Differential	%			
Neutrophils	54–62			
Lymphocytes	20–40			
Monocytes	3–7			
Eosinophils	1–3			
Basophils	0–1		*Low*	• Viral infection • Aplastic anemia • Chemotherapy
Platelets	150,000–350,000/mm³ or μl	200–400 × 10⁹/L	*High*	• Hemorrhage • Infections • Malignancy • Splenectomy
			Low	• Aplastic anemia • Chemotherapy • Hypersplenism

Coagulation Tests*

	Conventional Units	SI Units	Implications	
Bleeding time (template method)	2.75–8.0 min	2.75–8.0 min	*Prolonged*	• Aspirin ingestion • Low platelet count
Coagulation time	5–15 min	5–15 min	*Prolonged*	• Heparin therapy
Prothrombin time (PT)	12–14 sec	12–14 sec	*Prolonged*	• Vitamin K deficiency • Hepatic disease • Oral anticoagulant therapy

* From Chabner D-E: The Language of Medicine, 7th ed. Philadelphia, WB Saunders, 2004.

Red Blood Cell Tests*

	Conventional Units	SI Units	Implications
Hematocrit (Hct)			
Females	37%–47%	0.37–0.47	*High* • Polycythemia
Males	40%–54%	0.40–0.54	• Dehydration
			Low • Loss of blood
			• Anemia
Hemoglobin (Hgb)			
Females	12.0–14.0 gm/dL	1.86–2.48 mmol/L	*High* • Polycythemia
Males	14.0–16.0 gm/dL	2.17–2.79 mmol/L	• Dehydration
			Low • Anemia
			• Blood loss

* From Chabner D-E: The Language of Medicine, 7th ed. Philadelphia, WB Saunders, 2004.

Serum Tests*

	Conventional Units	SI Units	Implications	
Alanine aminotransferase (ALT, SGPT)	5–30 U/L	5–30 U/L	High	• Hepatitis
Albumin	3.5–5.5 gm/dL	35–55 g/L	Low	• Hepatic disease • Malnutrition • Nephritis and nephrosis
Alkaline phosphatase (ALP)	20–90 U/L	20–90 U/L	High	• Bone disease • Hepatitis or tumor infiltration of liver • Biliary obstruction
Aspartate aminotransferase (AST, SGOT)	10–30 U/L	10–30 U/L	High	• Hepatitis • Cardiac and muscle injury

*From Chabner D-E: The Language of Medicine, 7th ed. Philadelphia, WB Saunders, 2004.

Chart continued on following page

Serum Tests *Continued*

	Conventional Units	SI Units	Implications
Bilirubin			
Total	0.3–1.0 mg/dL	5.1–1.7 μmol/L	*High* • Hemolysis • Neonatal hepatic immaturity
Neonates	1–12 mg/dL	17–205 μmol/L	• Cirrhosis • Biliary tract obstruction
Blood urea nitrogen (BUN)	10–20 mg/dL	3.6–7.1 mmol/L	*High* • Renal disease • Reduced renal blood flow • Urinary tract obstruction *Low* • Hepatic damage • Malnutrition
Calcium	9.0–10.5 mg/dL	2.2–2.6 mmol/L	*High* • Hyperparathyroidism • Multiple myeloma • Metastatic cancer *Low* • Hypoparathyroidism • Total parathyroidectomy

Serum Tests *Continued*

	Conventional Units	SI Units	Implications	
Cholesterol (desirable range)				
Total	<200 mg/dL	<5.2 mmol/L	*High*	• High fat diet
LDL cholesterol	<130 mg/dL	<3.36 mmol/L		• Inherited hypercholesterolemia
HDL cholesterol	>60 mg/dL	>1.55 mmol/L	*Low*	• Starvation
Creatine phosphokinase (CK)				
Females	30–135 U/L	30–135 U/L	*High*	• Myocardial infarction
Males	55–170 U/L	55–170 U/L		• Muscle disease
Creatinine	<1.5 mg/dL	<133 μmol/L	*High*	• Renal disease
Glucose (fasting)	75–115 mg/dL	4.2–6.4 mmol/L	*High*	• Diabetes mellitus
				• Hyperinsulinism
			Low	• Fasting
				• Hypothyroidism
				• Addison disease
				• Pituitary insufficiency

Chart continued on following page

231

Serum Tests *Continued*

	Conventional Units	SI Units	Implications	
Lactate dehydrogenase (LDH)	100–190 U/L	100–190 U/L	*High*	• Tissue necrosis • Lymphomas • Muscle disease
Phosphate (–PO$_4$)	3.0–4.5 mg/dL	1.0–1.5 mmol/L	*High*	• Renal failure • Bone metastases • Hypoparathyroidism
			Low	• Malnutrition • Malabsorption • Hyperparathyroidism
Potassium (K)	3.5–5.0 mEq/L	3.5–5.0 mmol/L	*High*	• Burn victims • Renal failure • Diabetic ketoacidosis
			Low	• Cushing syndrome • Loss of body fluids

Serum Tests *Continued*

	Conventional Units	SI Units	Implications	
Sodium (Na)	136–145 mEq/L	136–145 mmol/L	*High*	• Inadequate water intake • Water loss in excess of sodium
			Low	• Adrenal insufficiency • Inadequate sodium intake • Excessive sodium loss
Thyroxine (T₄)	5–12 µg/dL	64–154 nmol/L	*High*	• Graves disease (hyperthyroidism)
			Low	• Hypothyroidism
Uric acid			*High*	• Gout
Females	2.5–8.0 mg/dL	150–480 µmol/L		• Leukemia
Males	1.5–6.0 mg/dL	90–360 µmol/L		

Internet Resource*

Patient education is a serious responsibility for health care professionals. Many health care facilities develop their own patient teaching materials. There are also groups, associations, businesses, and agencies that develop patient education materials for dissemination to the public. There are many tools that can be used to improve an individual's knowledge about a particular health care problem or issue. These include, but are not limited to, pamphlets, movies, video tapes, audio tapes, newsletters, and computerized instruction. Information can also be supplied to the health care professional to develop materials. The names and addresses identified below are potential sources of information that have provided information for the Miller-Keane Encyclopedia and Dictionary of Medicine, Nursing, and Allied Health. Local chapters of national organizations may also be found in the telephone directory and may serve as valuable resources for patient education material. Encyclopedias and directories of health-related associations are an additional source of information or contacts.

Alcoholics Anonymous
PO Box 549
Grand Central Station
New York, NY 10163
Phone: 212-870-3400
Fax: 212-870-3003
Website: http://www.alcoholics-anonymous.org
Alcoholics Anonymous (AA) is a fellowship of sober alcoholics that collects no dues or fees. It is an unaffiliated, self-supporting fellowship that receives no outside funds. Its primary purpose is to carry the AA message to alcoholics who still suffer.

---

*From Miller-Keane: Encyclopedia & Dictionary of Medicine, Nursing, & Allied Health, 7th ed. Philadelphia, WB Saunders, 2004.

Alzheimer's Disease Education & Referral Center (ADEAR)
PO Box 8250
Silver Spring, MD 20907-8250
Phone: 800-438-4380
Fax: 301-495-3334
Email: adear@alzheimers.org
Website: http://www.alzheimers.org

The Center provides information about Alzheimer's disease, its symptoms and diagnosis, and Alzheimer's disease research supported by the National Institute on Aging. It offers a newsletter to health professionals and other free publications to the public. Information specialists will answer questions about Alzheimer's disease by email.

Alzheimer Society of Canada
20 Eglinton Avenue W., Suite 1200
Toronto, ON M4R 1K8
Phone: 416-488-8772
Toll-free: 800-616-8816 (valid in Canada only)
Fax: 416-488-3778
Email: info@alzheimer.ca
Website: http://www.alzheimer.ca

The Society is a national voluntary organization whose goals are to provide information and support to those affected by Alzheimer's disease and their families, to increase public awareness of Alzheimer's disease, and to search for a cause and a cure.

American Association for Homecare
625 Slaters Lane, Suite 200
Alexandria, VA 22314-1171
Phone: 703-836-6263
Fax: 703-836-6730
Website: http://www.aahomecare.org

The American Association for Homecare (AAHomecare) is the unified voice that represents all the elements of home care under one roof—from home medical equipment and respiratory therapy to home health services and from rehabilitation technology to infusion therapy. AAHomecare is dedicated to working to advance the value and practice of quality health care services at home.

American Council of the Blind
1155 15th Street NW, Suite 720
Washington, DC 20005
Phone: 202-467-5081
Toll-free: 800-424-8666
Fax: 202-467-5085
Website: http://www.acb.org
The American Council of the Blind is a national membership organization established to promote independence, dignity, and well-being of blind and visually impaired people. Services include a monthly magazine, the Braille Forum, subscriptions to which are available free of charge to individuals in the US in Braille, large print, cassettes, and 3.5 DOS diskettes.

American Dietetic Association
216 West Jackson Boulevard
Chicago, IL 60606
Phone: 312-899-0040
Toll-free: 800-366-1655 (Consumer Hotline)
Website: http://www.eatright.org
The American Dietetic Association (ADA) promotes the optimal health, nutrition, and well-being of the public. The National Center for Nutrition and Dietetics maintains a consumer nutrition hotline that provides information and referrals to registered dietitians throughout the country.

Amyotrophic Lateral Sclerosis (ALS) Association
ALS Association National Office
27001 Agoura Road, Suite 150
Calabasas Hills, CA 91301-5104
Information and Referral Service: 800-782-4747
All others: 818-880-9007
Website: http://www.alsa.org
The mission of ALS Association is to discover the cause and cure for amyotrophic lateral sclerosis (Lou

Gehrig disease) through dedicated research while providing patient support, information and education for health care professionals and the general public, and advocacy for ALS research and health care concerns.

Association of Community Cancer Centers
1600 Nebel Street, Suite 201
Rockville, MD 20852
Phone: 301-984-9496
Fax: 301-770-1949
Website: http://www.accc-cancer.org
The mission of the Association of Community Cancer Centers is to promote the continuum of quality cancer care (research, prevention, screening, early detection, diagnosis, treatment, psychosocial services, rehabilitation, and hospice) for patients with cancer and the community.

Asthma and Allergy Foundation of America (AAFA)
1233 20th Street NW, Suite 402
Washington, DC 20036
Phone: 202-466-7943
Fax: 202-466-8940
Website: http://www.aafa.org
AAFA has been in existence for over 40 years and is a registered not-for-profit patient education organization dedicated to finding a cure for and controlling asthma and allergic diseases.

Bulimia Anorexia Nervosa Association (BANA)
300 Cabana Road East
Windsor, ON N9G 1A3
Phone: 519-969-2112
Fax: 519-969-0227
Email: info@bana.ca
Website: http://www.bana.ca
The objectives of BANA are to eradicate eating disorders; to promote healthy eating and acceptance of diverse body shapes; and to provide clinical, preventive, and advocacy services for people affected by eating disorders.

Canada Safety Council
1020 Thomas Spratt Place
Ottawa, ON K1G 5L5
Phone: 613-739-1535
Fax: 613-739-1566
Email: csc@safety-council.org
Website: http://www.safety-council.org
The Canada Safety Council is Canada's national not-for-profit safety organization. Its mission is to be a leader in the effort to reduce preventable deaths, injuries, and economic loss in traffic, work, home, community, and leisure environments.

Canadian Cystic Fibrosis Foundation
2221 Yonge Street, Suite 601
Toronto, ON M4S 2B4
Phone: 416-485-9149
Toll free (from Canada only): 800-378-2233
Fax: 416-485-0960
Website: http://www.cysticfibrosis.ca
The purpose and objectives of the Canadian Cystic Fibrosis Foundation are to aid those afflicted with cystic fibrosis; to conduct research in improved care and treatment and seek a cure or control for cystic fibrosis; to promote public awareness through the dissemination of information using all forms of communication; and to raise funds and allocate same for the above purposes.

Canadian Hard of Hearing Association (CHHA)
2435 Holly Lane, Suite 205
Ottawa, ON K1V 7P2
Voice Phone: 613-526-1584
TTY: 613-526-2692
Toll-free: 800-263-8068
Fax: 613-526-4718
Website: http://www.chha.ca
The Canadian Hard of Hearing Association is the "voice" of the hard of hearing in Canada. CHHA is the only Canadian national nonprofit consumer organization run by and for hard of hearing people. CHHA

exists to help the hard of hearing achieve independent, productive, and fulfilling lives.

Canadian Mental Health Association
2160 Yonge Street, Third Floor
Toronto, ON M4S 2Z3
Phone: 416-484-7750
Fax: 416-484-4617
Website: http://www.cmha.ca
The Canadian Mental Health Association is a national voluntary association that exists to promote mental health. CMHA's mission is operationalized through education, advocacy, research, service provision, and facilitation.

Canadian National Institute for the Blind (CNIB)
1929 Bayview Avenue
Toronto, ON M4G 3E8
Phone: 416-486-2500
Email: cnib@icomm.ca
Website: http://www.icomm.ca/cnib/
CNIB is the world's largest provider of services to people with visual impairments and a global leader in adaptive and assistive technologies.

Cancer Care, Inc.
275 7th Avenue
New York, NY 10001
Phone: 800-813-HOPE
Website: http://www.cancercare.org
Offers information, referral, individual and group counseling, and patient education free of charge.

Centers for Disease Control and Prevention (CDC)
1600 Clifton Road, NE
Atlanta, GA 30333
Phone: 800-311-3435
Website: http://www.cdc.gov
The CDC provides information on diseases, health risks, prevention guidelines, and strategies. A wide variety of services can be accessed through the CDC.

Clinical Reference Systems, Ltd.
335 Interlocken Parkway
Broomfield, CO 80021
Phone: 800-237-8401
Fax: 303-460-6282
Website: http://www.patienteducation.com
Contact: Sales Department
Clinical Reference Systems, Ltd. (CRS) offers software designed to generate patient education handouts in Windows and web-based formats in a wide variety of areas. Editing of topics and customizing of handouts are features.

The Combined Health Information Database (CHID)
7830 Old Georgetown Road
Bethesda, MD 20814
Website: http://chid.nih.gov
CHID is a cooperative effort among several federal agencies of the United States government. These agencies have combined their information files into one database, which has been available to the public since 1985. Topics are updated four times per year.

Crohn's and Colitis Foundation of Canada (CCFC)
60 St. Clair Avenue East, Suite 600
Toronto, ON M4T 1N5
Phone: 416-920-5035
Toll-free (from Canada only): 800-387-1479
Fax: 416-929-0364
Website: http://www.ccfc.ca
The CCFC is a national not-for-profit voluntary foundation dedicated to finding the cure for Crohn's disease and ulcerative colitis. To realize this the CCFC is committed to raising increasing funds for research. The CCFC also believes that it is important to make all individuals with inflammatory bowel disease aware of the Foundation, and to educate these individuals, their families, health professionals, and the general public.

Cystic Fibrosis Foundation
6931 Arlington Road
Bethesda, MD 20814
Phone: 301-951-4422
Toll-free: 800-344-4823
Fax: 301-951-6378
Email: info@cff.org
Website: http://www.cff.org

The Cystic Fibrosis Foundation was established in 1955 to raise money to fund research to find a cure for cystic fibrosis and to improve the quality of life for the 30,000 children and adults with the disease.

Endometriosis Association
International Headquarters
8585 N. 76th Place
Milwaukee, WI 53223
Phone: 414-355-2200
Fax: 414-355-6065
Toll-free: 800-992-3636
Website: http://www.endometriosisassn.org

The Endometriosis Association is a self-help organization dedicated to offering support and information to women with endometriosis, educating the public and medical community about the disease, and promoting and conducting research related to endometriosis.

Epilepsy Foundation
4321 Garden City Drive
Landover, MD 20785
Phone: 301-459-3700
Toll-free: 800-EFA-1000
Website: http://www.epilepsyfoundation.org

The Epilepsy Foundation is the national organization that works for people affected by seizures through research, education, advocacy, and service.

International Federation on Ageing (IFA)
380 Rue Saint-Antoine Ouest, Bureau 3200
Montreal, PQ H2Y 3X7
Phone: 514-287-9679
Website: http://www.ifa-fiv.org

IFA serves as an advocate for the well-being of older persons around the world. IFA is committed to providing a worldwide forum on aging issues and concerns and to fostering the development of associations and agencies that serve or represent older persons.

La Leche League Canada
Box 29, 18C Industrial Drive
Chesterville, ON K0C 1H0
Phone: 613-448-1842
Fax: 613-448-1845
Website: http://www.lalecheleaguecanada.ca
La Leche League Canada promotes a better understanding of breastfeeding as an important element in the healthy development of the baby, and through education, information, encouragement, and mother-to-mother support helps mothers nationwide to breastfeed. The main objective of La Leche League Canada is to help mothers breastfeed their babies.

Learning Disabilities Association of America
4156 Library Road
Pittsburgh, PA 15234
Phone: 412-341-1515
Fax: 412-344-0224
Email: info@ldaamerica.org
Website: http://www.ldanatl.org
LDA is an information and referral organization. The Association provides any and all information regarding learning disabilities in both children and adults. There are 500 chapters across the country. Once individuals make contact with LDA, the Association provides a free packet of material, then refers them to one of the Association's chapters. Membership is also offered.

National Asian Pacific Center on Aging
1511 Third Avenue, Suite 914
Seattle, WA 98121
Phone: 206-624-1221
Fax: 206-624-1023
Website: http://www.napca.org

The National Asian Pacific Center on Aging (NAPCA) is the leading advocacy organization committed to the well-being of elderly Asians and Pacific Islanders in the United States. NAPCA develops and administers programs to enhance the dignity and quality of life of its constituents. NAPCA provides a fax-on-demand service for over 300 pamphlets, brochures, fact sheets, etc. in 15 languages on topics related to health, wellness, and social services. FAX-IT can be reached by dialing 206-624-0185 from any fax machine (telephone handset).

National Association for Visually Handicapped
22 West 21st Street
New York, NY 10010
Phone: 212-255-2804
Fax: 212-727-2931
Website: http://www.navh.org
The Association's primary goal is to promote hope, dignity, and productivity for those with uncorrectable visual impairments by encouraging the full use of residual vision through large print, visual aids, emotional support, educational outreach, advocacy, and referral services.

National Cancer Institute Information Associates Program
9300 Old Georgetown Road
Bethesda, MD 20814-1519
Phone: 301-496-7600
Toll-free: 800-624-7890
The Program provides access to the National Cancer Institute's information resources for health professionals, including the journal of the National Cancer Institute.

National Clearinghouse for Alcohol & Drug Information (NCADI)
11426 Rockville Pike, Suite 200
Rockville, MD 20852-3007
Phone: 800-729-6686
TDD: 800-487-4889
Fax: 301-468-6433
Website: http://www.health.org

A service of the US Center for Substance Abuse Prevention, NCADI collects and distributes information about alcohol, tobacco, and other drugs to all interested persons. The Clearinghouse provides a wide variety of free printed material as well as video tapes and disk-based products for a small cost-recovery fee.

National Clearinghouse on Child Abuse and Neglect Information
PO Box 1182
Washington, DC 20013-1182
Phone: 800-394-3366
Fax: 703-385-3206
Website: http://www.calib.com/nccanch
The Clearinghouse collects, catalogues, stores, organizes, and disseminates information on all aspects of child maltreatment.

National Committee for the Prevention of Elder Abuse
101 Vermont Avenue NW, Suite 1001
Washington, DC 20002
Phone: 202-682-4140
Fax: 202-682-3984
Website: http://www.preventelderabuse.org
The National Committee for the Prevention of Elder Abuse was established to promote greater understanding of elder abuse and the development of services to protect older persons and disabled adults and reduce the likelihood of their being abused, neglected, and/or exploited.

National Council on Alcoholism and Drug Dependence, Inc.
21 Exchange Place, Suite 2902
New York, NY 10005
Phone: 212-269-7797
Website: http://www.ncadd.org
The National Council on Alcoholism and Drug Dependence, Inc. (NCADD) provides education, information, help, and hope in the fight against the chronic

and often fatal disease of alcoholism and other drug addictions. Founded in 1944, NCADD, with its nation-wide network of affiliates, advocates prevention, intervention, and treatment, and is committed to ridding the disease of its stigma and its sufferers of their denial and shame.

National Health Council
1730 M Street NW, Suite 500
Washington, DC 20036
Phone: 202-785-3910
Fax: 202-785-5923
Email: info@nationalhealthcouncil.org
Website: http://www.nationalhealthcouncil.org
The National Health Council is a private, nonprofit association of national organizations that was founded in 1920 as a clearinghouse and cooperative effort for voluntary health agencies (VHAs).

National Institute of Nutrition (NIN)
265 Carling Avenue, Suite 302
Ottawa, ON K1S 2E11
Phone: 613-235-3355
Website: http://www.nin.ca
Founded in 1983, NIN is a private, nonprofit national organization dedicated to bridging the gap between the science and practice of nutrition and serving as a credible source of information on nutrition. The NIN also conducts and supports nutrition research.

National Wellness Institute, Inc.
1300 College Court
PO Box 827
Stevens Point, WI 54481-0827
Phone: 715-342-2969
Fax: 715-342-2979
Website: http://www.nationalwellness.org
National Wellness Institute, Inc. has served profes-sionals interested in wellness and health promotion since 1977. It focuses on professional education pro-grams; resources and information dissemination

through its professional association, the National Wellness Association; and the development and distribution of lifestyle inventories and health risk appraisals.

The Nemours Foundation
The Alfred I. duPont Institute
1600 Rockland Road
Wilmington, DE 19803
Website: http://www.kidshealth.org
The Foundation maintains a very informative website known as KidsHealth.

Osteoporosis Society of Canada
33 Laird Drive
Toronto, ON M5S 3A7
Phone: 416-696-2817
Toll-free (from Canada only): 800-463-6842
Website: http://www.osteoporosis.ca
The Society educates and empowers individuals and communities in the prevention and treatment of osteoporosis. It is a resource for patients, health professionals, the media, and the general public who seek medically accurate information on the causes, prevention, and treatment of osteoporosis.

Pregnancy and Infant Loss Center
1421 East Wayzata Boulevard #30
Wayzata, MN 55391
The Pregnancy and Infant Loss Center is a national nonprofit organization, founded in 1983, providing support, resources, and education on miscarriage, stillbirth, and infant death.

SHARE Pregnancy & Infant Loss Support, Inc.
National Office
St. Joseph Health Center
300 First Capitol Drive
St. Charles, MO 63301
Phone: 800-821-6819
Fax: 314-947-7486
Website: http://www.nationalshareoffice.com

SHARE offers support to families and caregivers whose lives have been touched by the tragic death of a baby through miscarriage, stillbirth, or newborn death by providing information, education, and a network of support groups across the country.

Recording for the Blind and Dyslexic (RFB & D)
20 Roszel Road
Princeton, NJ 08540
Phone: 609-452-0606
Toll-free: 800-221-4792
Website: http://www.rfbd.org
RFB & D maintains the world's largest collection of professional resources and textbooks on audio tape for all academic levels. It serves people who cannot read standard print because of a visual, perceptual, or other physical disability.

SIECUS (Sexuality Information and Education Council of the United States)
Publication Department
130 West 42nd Street, Suite 350
New York, NY 10036-7802
Phone: 212-819-9770
Website: http://www.siecus.org
SIECUS affirms that sexuality is a natural and healthy part of living. SIECUS develops, collects, and disseminates information, promotes comprehensive education about sexuality, and advocates the right of individuals to make responsible sexual choices.

Students Against Destructive Decisions (SADD)
255 Main Street
PO Box 800
Marlborough, MA 01752
Phone: 877-SADD-INC
Fax: 508-481-5759
Website: http://www.saddonline.com
Founded as Students Against Driving Drunk, the organization provides young people with the tools to address the problems of underage drinking, impaired driving, drug use, and their consequences.

United Network for Organ Sharing (UNOS)
1100 Boulders Parkway, Suite 500
Richmond, VA 23225
Phone: 804-330-8500
Website: http://www.unos.org

UNOS, under contract with the US Department of Health and Human Services, is a nonprofit organization that administers the National Organ Procurement and Transplantation Network (OPTN) and the US Scientific Registry of Organ Transplant Recipients mandated by Congress. It operates and maintains the national list of patients waiting for solid organ transplants. In addition, it maintains a computer-assisted system for allocating organs to individuals on the waiting list. The primary goal of the UNOS organization is to increase the number of donated organs. Through a number of strategies, including public and professional education, UNOS endeavors to bridge the gap between the number of individuals waiting for transplant and the number of organs donated.

Information about organ donation and transplantation is available from UNOS 24 hours a day, 365 days a year.

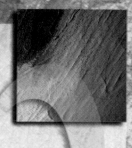

part 3

BODY SYSTEMS
ILLUSTRATIONS*

*Illustrations modified from Chabner D-E: The
Language of Medicine, 7th ed. Philadelphia,
WB Saunders, 2004; Miller-Keane: Encyclopedia &
Dictionary of Medicine, Nursing, & Allied Health,
7th ed. Philadelphia, WB Saunders, 2003.

Index of Body Systems Illustrations

This is an index of all the important labels in the following illustrations of the body systems. You can use it to locate the relevant illustration for a particular anatomical term you may have in mind.

THE CARDIOVASCULAR SYSTEM
(AORTA AND MAJOR ARTERIES)

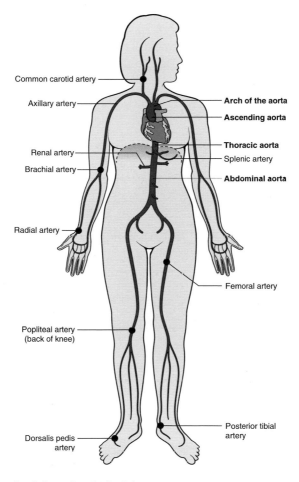

Common carotid artery

Axillary artery

Renal artery

Brachial artery

Radial artery

Popliteal artery
(back of knee)

Dorsalis pedis
artery

Arch of the aorta

Ascending aorta

Thoracic aorta

Splenic artery

Abdominal aorta

Femoral artery

Posterior tibial
artery

Dots indicate pulse points in arteries

THE CARDIOVASCULAR SYSTEM (HEART)

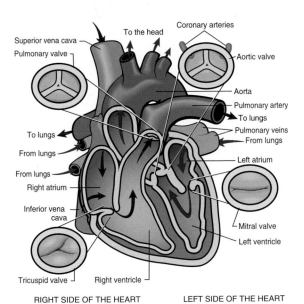

Superior vena cava

Pulmonary valve

To the head

Coronary arteries

Aortic valve

Aorta

Pulmonary artery

To lungs

To lungs

From lungs

Pulmonary veins

From lungs

From lungs

Left atrium

Right atrium

Inferior vena cava

Mitral valve

Left ventricle

Tricuspid valve

Right ventricle

RIGHT SIDE OF THE HEART   LEFT SIDE OF THE HEART

THE DIGESTIVE SYSTEM

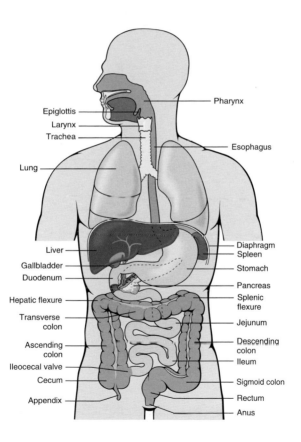

Epiglottis
Larynx
Trachea
Lung
Liver
Gallbladder
Duodenum
Hepatic flexure
Transverse colon
Ascending colon
Ileocecal valve
Cecum
Appendix

Pharynx
Esophagus
Diaphragm
Spleen
Stomach
Pancreas
Splenic flexure
Jejunum
Descending colon
Ileum
Sigmoid colon
Rectum
Anus

THE EAR

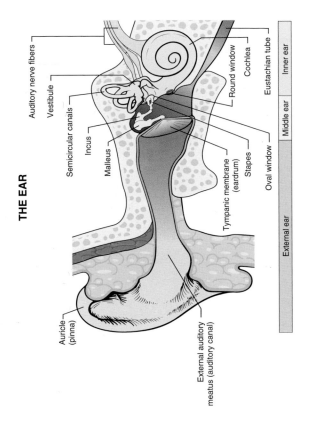

- Auricle (pinna)
- External auditory meatus (auditory canal)
- Auditory nerve fibers
- Vestibule
- Semicircular canals
- Incus
- Malleus
- Tympanic membrane (eardrum)
- Stapes
- Oval window
- Round window
- Cochlea
- Eustachian tube

| External ear | Middle ear | Inner ear |

THE ENDOCRINE SYSTEM

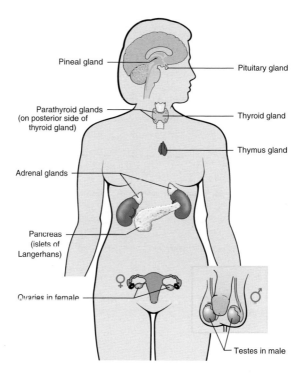

Pineal gland

Pituitary gland

Parathyroid glands
(on posterior side of
thyroid gland)

Thyroid gland

Thymus gland

Adrenal glands

Pancreas
(islets of
Langerhans)

Ovaries in female

Testes in male

THE EYE

- Conjunctiva
- Cornea
- Lens
- Pupil
- Path of light
- Anterior chamber
- Iris
- Ciliary body
- Retina
- Optic disc
- Optic nerve
- Fovea centralis
- Macula
- Choroid layer
- Sclera
- Vitreous humor

THE INTEGUMENTARY SYSTEM (SKIN)

Stratum corneum
Keratinized (horny) cells
Basal layer
Melanocytes

Dermis

B

Epidermis
Dermis
Subcutaneous tissue

Nerve ending
Sebaceous gland
Sweat gland
Hair follicle
Hair root
Blood vessels

A

THE LYMPHATIC SYSTEM

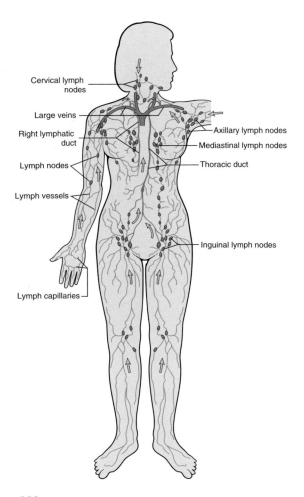

Cervical lymph nodes

Large veins

Right lymphatic duct

Lymph nodes

Lymph vessels

Lymph capillaries

Axillary lymph nodes

Mediastinal lymph nodes

Thoracic duct

Inguinal lymph nodes

THE ANTERIOR SUPERFICIAL MUSCLES

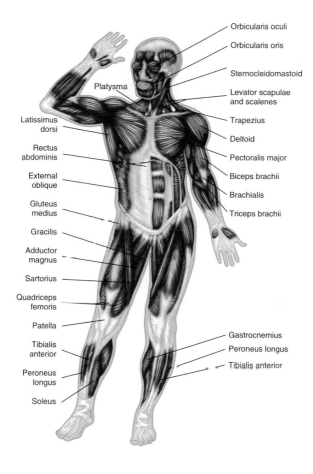

Orbicularis oculi

Orbicularis oris

Sternocleidomastoid

Levator scapulae
and scalenes

Platysma

Trapezius

Latissimus
dorsi

Deltoid

Rectus
abdominis

Pectoralis major

External
oblique

Biceps brachii

Brachialis

Gluteus
medius

Triceps brachii

Gracilis

Adductor
magnus

Sartorius

Quadriceps
femoris

Patella

Gastrocnemius

Tibialis
anterior

Peroneus longus

Peroneus
longus

Tibialis anterior

Soleus

THE POSTERIOR SUPERFICIAL MUSCLES

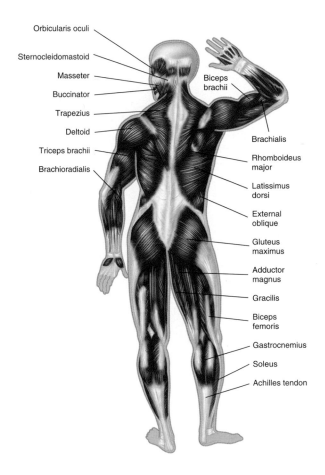

Orbicularis oculi

Sternocleidomastoid

Masseter

Buccinator

Trapezius

Deltoid

Triceps brachii

Brachioradialis

Biceps brachii

Brachialis

Rhomboideus major

Latissimus dorsi

External oblique

Gluteus maximus

Adductor magnus

Gracilis

Biceps femoris

Gastrocnemius

Soleus

Achilles tendon

THE NERVOUS SYSTEM

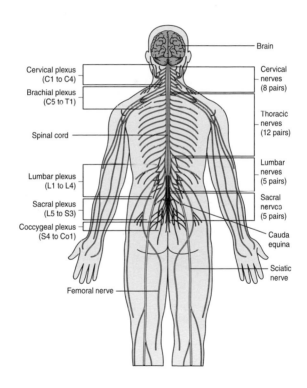

Brain

Cervical plexus
(C1 to C4)

Brachial plexus
(C5 to T1)

Spinal cord

Lumbar plexus
(L1 to L4)

Sacral plexus
(L5 to S3)

Coccygeal plexus
(S4 to Co1)

Femoral nerve

Cervical
nerves
(8 pairs)

Thoracic
nerves
(12 pairs)

Lumbar
nerves
(5 pairs)

Sacral
nerves
(5 pairs)

Cauda
equina

Sciatic
nerve

THE FEMALE REPRODUCTIVE SYSTEM

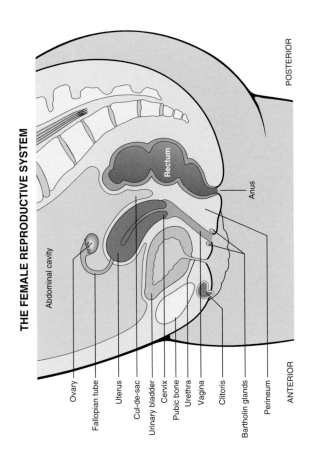

POSTERIOR

Abdominal cavity

Rectum

Anus

Ovary

Fallopian tube

Uterus

Cul-de-sac

Urinary bladder

Cervix

Pubic bone

Urethra

Vagina

Clitoris

Bartholin glands

Perineum

ANTERIOR

THE MALE REPRODUCTIVE SYSTEM

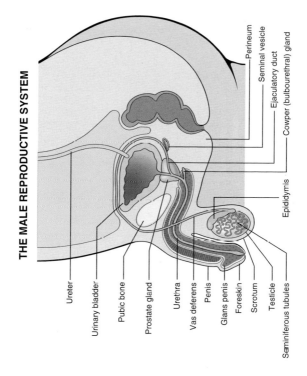

- Ureter
- Urinary bladder
- Pubic bone
- Prostate gland
- Urethra
- Vas deferens
- Penis
- Glans penis
- Foreskin
- Scrotum
- Testicle
- Seminiferous tubules
- Perineum
- Seminal vesicle
- Ejaculatory duct
- Cowper (bulbourethral) gland
- Epididymis

THE RESPIRATORY SYSTEM

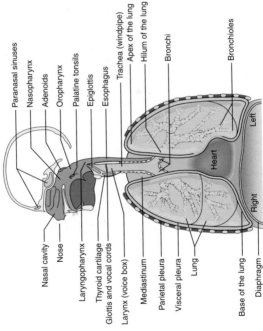

Paranasal sinuses
Nasopharynx
Adenoids
Oropharynx
Palatine tonsils
Epiglottis
Esophagus
Trachea (windpipe)
Apex of the lung
Hilum of the lung
Bronchi
Bronchioles

Nasal cavity
Nose
Laryngopharynx
Thyroid cartilage
Glottis and vocal cords
Larynx (voice box)
Mediastinum
Parietal pleura
Visceral pleura
Lung
Base of the lung
Diaphragm

Heart
Left
Right

THE SKELETAL SYSTEM

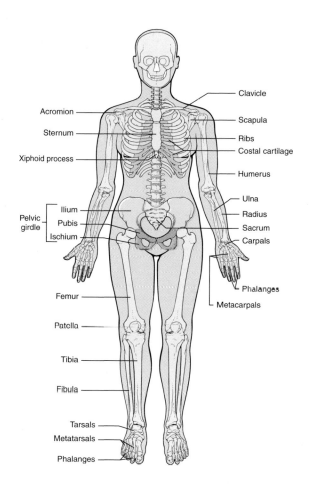

Clavicle

Acromion

Scapula

Sternum

Ribs

Costal cartilage

Xiphoid process

Humerus

Ulna

Ilium

Radius

Pelvic girdle

Pubis

Sacrum

Ischium

Carpals

Phalanges

Femur

Metacarpals

Patella

Tibia

Fibula

Tarsals

Metatarsals

Phalanges

THE URINARY SYSTEM

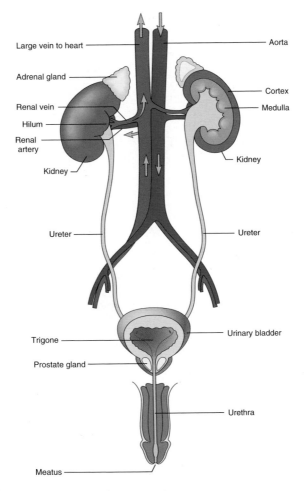

Large vein to heart

Adrenal gland

Renal vein

Hilum

Renal artery

Kidney

Ureter

Trigone

Prostate gland

Meatus

Aorta

Cortex

Medulla

Kidney

Ureter

Urinary bladder

Urethra